Preface

This section starts appropriately in considering the principles which should govern our care of the injured child and the background factors which influence fracture epidemiology. Knowing how to manage the multiply injured child and recognizing the one who has been non-accidentally injured are essential skills in our specialty. Injuries to the growth plate are not always easy to recognize and manage but, if we fail to do so, the long-term consequences may be serious. Succeeding chapters describe childhood injuries and fractures regionally. Conservative fracture management has not been forgotten amidst the plethora of newer methods of surgical fixation.

Michael KD Benson, Oxford, UK   John A Fixsen, London, UK
Malcolm F Macnicol, Edinburgh, UK   Klaus Parsch, Stuttgart, Germany

June, 2011

Children's Upper and Lower Limb Fractures

Michael Benson • John Fixsen • Malcolm Macnicol
Klaus Parsch
Editors

Children's Upper and Lower Limb Fractures

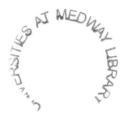

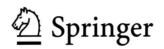

Editors

Michael Benson
Ridgway
Harberton Mead
OX3 ODB Oxford
United Kingdom
michael.benson@doctors.org.uk

John Fixsen
West Barn
Clamok Farm Barns
Wier Quay
PL20 7BU Bere Alston
United Kingdom
jafixsen@btinternet.com

Malcolm Macnicol
Red House
Gillsland Road 1
EH10 5DE Edinburgh
United Kingdom
mmacnicol@aol.com

Klaus Parsch
Weinbergweg 68
70569 Stuttgart Baden-
Württemberg
Germany
kparsch@t-online.de

ISBN 978-0-85729-554-5   e-ISBN 978-0-85729-555-2
DOI 10.1007/978-0-85729-555-2
Springer London Dordrecht Heidelberg New York

British Library Cataloguing in Publication Data
A catalogue record for this book is available from the British Library

Library of Congress Control Number: 2011929880

Cover design: eStudio Calamar S.L.

Printed on acid-free paper

Springer is part of Springer Science+Business Media (www.springer.com)

Foreword

Confirming the British genetic trait for writing and publishing (as well as acting), two English (Oxford and London) and a Scottish orthopaedic surgeon (Edinburgh) have produced a third edition of their comprehensive text, joined, as in the second edition by an editor from Germany, recognizing its part in the European community. The 62 physician contributors are drawn from pink-colored countries in our childhood geography books—the old British Empire from Australia to Zambia and two from the former colony, the USA.

The original purpose of the book was to give residents or registrars an easily accessible and concise description of diseases and conditions encountered in the practice of paediatric orthopaedic surgery and to prepare for their examinations. But the practicing orthopaedic surgeon will find an update of current practice that can be read for clarity and constraint—enough but not too much. A foreword might be a preview of things to come, but a "back word" of what was thought to be the final say on the subject is needed for a perspective in progress.

A "back word" look reveals the tremendous progress in medical diagnosis and treatment of which paediatric orthopaedics and fracture care is a component. Clubfoot treatment based on the dictums of Hiram Kite has had a revolutionary change by Ponseti. The chapter by Eastwood has the details on cast application and orthotics follow-up to obtain the 95% correction without the extensive surgery many of us thought was needed.

Paediatric fracture care has also changed from traction for fractures of the femoral shaft in the ages of 5–15 years to intramedullary fixation with elastic stable nails originated in Nancy and Metz, France—"Nancy nails." Klaus Parsch's chapter tells us that it is their preferred method of treatment in Stuttgart, Germany.

Robert Dickson's lucid writing on idiopathic scoliosis as primarily a rotation of the lordotic thoracic spine again bears study to deepen the understanding that it is a three-dimensional deformity. As in the past editions, a coat hanger helps to appreciate the distortion of curvatures in a one-dimensional radiograph. Those orthopaedists who need courage to resist pressure to encase children in casts or braces or orthoses will be heartened to know that none of these conservative measures have shown any effect in prevention or curve progression. What to do instead of "treatment"? Read on.

This is not a book to learn the details of surgical technique–other texts and only experience can do that. Even though a seasoned orthopaedic surgeon does not need this knowledge to pass an examination, he or she is expected to know something about the subject. Once identified as an orthopaedic surgeon, your opinion is often sought at social events usually standing with a drink in hand. And commonly it is advice sought by your married children about a grandchild's musculoskeletal problem. Can you answer sensibly? If, "I'll get back to you later" is your response, a quick perusal of the contents of this volume should help maintain your professional standing and as is now the fashion of school teachers, your "self-esteem." And you won't have to log on to the Internet.

Eugene E Bleck

Contents

Contributors

Franck Accadbled Hôpital des Enfants, Toulouse, France

Michael K. d'A. Benson Nuffield Orthopaedic Centre, Oxford, UK

Peter W. Engelhardt Department of Orthopedic Surgery, Hirslanden Clinic Aarau, Aarau, Switzerland

Francisco Fernandez Fernandez Department of Pediatric Orthopaedic Surgery, Olgahospital, Stuttgart, Germany

Bruce K. Foster Department of Orthopaedic Surgery, Women's and Children's Hospital, Adelaide, SA, Australia

Carol-C. Hasler Department of Orthopaedics, University Children's Hospital Basel, Basel, Switzerland

James B. Hunter Departments of Trauma and Orthopaedics, Nottingham University Hospital, Nottingham, UK

Lennart A. Landin Department of Orthopaedics, Malmö University Hospital, Malmö, Sweden

Malcolm F. Macnicol University of Edinburgh; Royal Hospital for Sick Children; Edinburgh and Murrayfield Hospital; Royal Infirmary; Edinburgh, UK

Jacqueline Y. Q. Mok Community Child Health Department, Royal Hospital for Sick Children, Edinburgh, UK

Alastair W. Murray Department of Children's Orthopaedics, Royal Hospital for Sick Children, Edinburgh, UK

Cathrin S. Parsch Emergency Department Lyell McEwin Health Services and Medstar Emergency Retrieval Services, Adelaide, South Australia, Australia

Klaus Parsch Orthopaedic Department, Pediatric Centre Olgahospital, Stuttgart, Germany

Peter P. Schmittenbecher Department of Pediatric Surgery, Municipal Hospital, Karlsruhe, Germany

Peter J. Witherow[†] Bristol Royal Hospital for Sick Children, Bristol, UK

Chapter 1

Principles of Fracture Care

Malcolm F. Macnicol and Alastair W. Murray

Introduction

In childhood, bone has certain characteristics that are qualitatively different from those of the adult. First, the modulus of elasticity is relatively high and the thick periosteal sleeve adds further resistance to complete fracturing. Hence buckle (torus) and greenstick fractures are relatively common, although they may be more extensive than plain radiographs suggest. Second, it should be appreciated that bone tends to give way before ligament in the prepubertal child: apophyses and other bony points of soft tissue attachment avulse before the tendon ruptures or the ligament tears.

The etiology of paediatric fractures is discussed by Landin (see Chapter 2) and Ibrahim and Abdul-Hamid (see Chapter 12 of General Principles of Children's Orthopaedic Disease); to some extent, it is culturally determined. The incidence of skeletal injury varies geographically and between urban and rural communities while increased social deprivation is associated with a greater likelihood of skeletal injury in childhood. In temperate countries, seasonal variations and alteration in the hours of daylight also affect fracture patterns. Epidemiological studies are important, as they identify trends and hazards and have led to significant improvements in child safety such as the mandatory use of child car seats in many countries and safer surfaces in play parks. In the first year of life, the frequency of fracturing is equivalent in the two sexes, but boys are twice as likely to fracture during late childhood and adolescence, just as they are more than twice as likely to die from severe injury. Pathological changes in the skeleton may predispose to fracture and are dealt with later in this chapter.

The psychological impact of trauma in childhood should also be considered. Anxiety and depression following accidents is well recognized in children of all ages and often not considered by clinicians [1]. Minimizing the stress of the hospital experience and having access to counseling for children and adults can be helpful.

Characteristics of Fractures

The sites of bony injury in the child differ from those in the adult, the most important difference relating to the fact that the bones of a child are actively growing. A paediatric fracture possesses greater potential to unite quickly and to remodel deformity. Whereas approximately one in six fractures are initially angulated more than 20° after reduction and splintage, 5 years after the injury this figure reduces to approximately 1 in 40. This capacity to realign depends principally upon the reorientation of the epiphysis and growth plate as the bone elongates.

In addition to the trophic changes in physeal growth (Fig. 1.1), which accounts for the majority of the correction, differential periosteal activity produces remodeling of the shaft, but does not supplement the growth realignment [2].

Successful remodeling of the malalignment is more likely

- in the younger child;
- the nearer the fracture is to the epiphyseal plate;
- if the deformity is angulated in the plane of the adjacent joint movement.

The history of growth and correction of malalignment is of interest. The monographs of Poland [3], Konig [4], Aitken [5], and Blount [6] recorded the pathophysiology of epiphyseal injury and the subsequent physeal response. The speed of correction is exponential rather than linear and appears to be the result of redistribution of loading through the growth plate. Little correction occurs if the primary angulation is

M.F. Macnicol (✉)
University of Edinburgh, Edinburgh, UK; Royal Hospital for Sick Children, Edinburgh, UK; Edinburgh and Murrayfield Hospital, Edinburgh, UK; Royal Infirmary, Edinburgh, UK

Fig. 1.1 The growth plate gradually realigns the epiphysis if anatomical reduction is not achieved. This process will not correct the deformity fully if the angulation is excessive

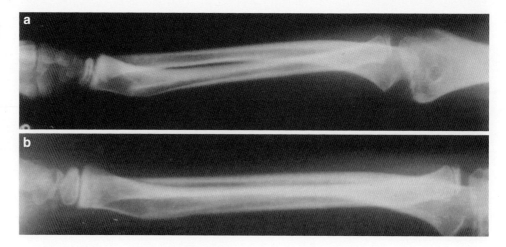

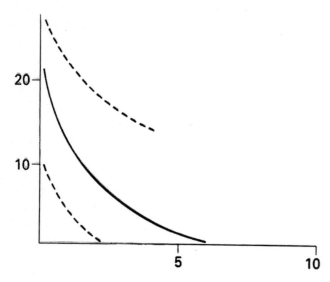

Fig. 1.2 Growth plate correction of malalignment is maximal in the first year, proceeding at a rate of approximately 1° per month (y-axis labeled "degrees of malalignment" and x-axis labeled "years")

less than 5°; in contrast, malalignment of more than 20° will usually not correct completely (Fig. 1.2). The correction is about 1 degree per month but the precise method of this trophic change is unknown. Pauwels [7] considered that increased pressure on the growth plate results in a stimulus to growth. This may explain the correction of genu varum in the toddler and the eventual lessening of valgus after a proximal tibial metaphyseal fracture. However, it is also known that longitudinal tension across the plate will decrease its growth rate, and Crilly [8] suggested that the periosteal sleeve may control axial growth by reining in the physis. Whatever the mechanism, the epiphysis tends to realign until it lies at 90° to the axial forces passing up the limb and this phenomenon is referred to as the Hueter–Volkmann principle.

Management

Management of the injured child must begin with the examining physician ensuring that life-threatening pathology has been successfully treated or excluded. The next priority is to prevent further damage to the soft tissues of the injured limb. Most importantly, this requires a prompt evaluation of the neurovascular integrity distal to the injury and early, effective action to alleviate ischemia or neuropathy. Urgent reduction of gross fracture displacement will usually restore an adequate blood supply if acute ischemia is encountered. If general anesthesia is likely to be delayed then it is quite appropriate to carry out a provisional reduction and splintage of a child's limb under sedation in the emergency department. The same applies when the degree of fracture displacement is leading to severe tenting of the soft tissues and blanching of the overlying skin. Undue delay in alleviating the pressure on the soft tissues will lead to soft tissue necrosis and possible skin breakdown at the fracture site. This is as true in children as it is in adults.

Early, adequate, and appropriate analgesia must be provided as this will lessen both the child's and the parent's distress and anxiety and make assessment easier. Intravenous opiate is often required for long bone fractures and early advice from colleagues expert in providing analgesia to children can be very useful. It should not be forgotten, however, that most fractures can be rendered significantly less painful by application of sufficient splintage at an early stage. Children with an unsupported fracture should not be made to wait for long periods for radiographs.

Open fractures in children require the same initial management as those encountered in the adult. Superficial lavage in the emergency department with removal of obvious, accessible contaminants is indicated. This should be followed by application of a sterile dressing which should then be left undisturbed until definitive treatment in the operating theater. The temptation to re-examine the wound prior to theater should be resisted as this increases the risk of infection and the distress of the child. The child's immunization status should be clarified and appropriate tetanus prophylaxis ensured. Administration of a broad spectrum, intravenous antibiotic should be carried out prior to leaving the emergency department. There is evidence that a delay of greater than 6 hours to definitive treatment of open fractures in children can be tolerated [9] but each case should be judged on its merits and rapid access to theater may be indicated in situations of severe soft tissue compromise. Adequate operative stabilization of significant open fractures should be the aim and can be achieved with internal or external fixation. Intramedullary stabilization of open diaphyseal fractures with titanium elastic nails appears to be safe and may have some advantages over external fixation [10]. The modified Gustilo classification (Table 1.1) [11] is often used to classify open fractures in children and has the benefit of facilitating a common understanding of the severity of a particular injury. It should be noted, however, that the Gustilo classification was developed from studying predominantly diaphyseal fractures in adults and, although commonly used, its prognostic value may not apply to children's fractures.

Compartment syndrome can develop in children and communication difficulties may lead to a delay in the diagnosis. Clinicians must be attentive for the cardinal symptom of increasing pain despite adequate immobilization and usual analgesia. Pain on passive stretching of involved muscles is a relatively early sign but development of altered sensation or circulation indicates that hypoxic damage to the compartment has been ongoing for some time [12]. Compartment pressure monitoring should be considered in children with high-risk fractures and impaired consciousness. Interpretation of the results is, however, hindered by the limited knowledge of normal values for children [13].

Effective management of musculoskeletal injury in children must also include early identification of conditions beyond local expertise or facilities. Early communication with a specialist center used to dealing with childhood injuries is recommended if any uncertainty exists.

Although paediatric fractures unite rapidly and are rarely associated with major complications, several management problems may be encountered. The young child, in particular, may be fretful and difficult to examine fully. Worried parents and a crying child pose problems for even the most experienced clinician.

Many fractures are difficult to see and therefore imaging must be of good quality. In addition to standard anteroposterior (AP) and lateral radiographs of the injured site, oblique views may be useful in cases of uncertainty. Reference to atlases of normal variants and the use of more advanced imaging has largely replaced the requirement for comparison radiographs of the opposite limb but this may still occasionally have a place. Computed tomography (CT) scans can provide highly detailed views of ossified tissue and are particularly useful in managing periarticular and complex physeal injuries. Magnetic resonance imaging (MRI) can aid in the diagnosis of osteochondral and soft tissue injury but is hampered by the frequent need to sedate or anesthetize the younger child.

Once a fracture has been identified, its site, degree of displacement, and the age of the patient determine whether reduction and possibly fixation are required. No firm prescription can be given in terms of acceptable angulation or malposition for defined age groups. However, as a general rule, mid-diaphyseal angulation of more than 10° is unacceptable, particularly in the older child. Rotational malalignment should be corrected fully but the overgrowth that follows long bone fracture may make a modest overlap at the fracture site desirable in some situations.

The three "*R*'s" of management are

1. realign the fracture
2. respect the soft tissues
3. remember the patient

These apply to children as much as to adults, although the alignment of long bone fractures can be slightly less precise and still allow good function ultimately.

Disruptions of the growth plate (physis) account for 15–20% of all paediatric fractures. This proportion is an underestimate because metaphyseal cracks may propagate

Table 1.1 Classification of open fractures [11]

Grade	Definition
1	Open fracture with a clean wound of less than 1 cm
2	Open fracture with a wound of greater than 1 cm but minimal soft tissue damage
3a	High-energy injury or heavily contaminated wound but with sufficient tissue to achieve soft tissue cover
3b	High-energy injury with periosteal stripping and bone exposure with insufficient soft tissue cover
3c	Any open fracture with limb threatening vascular injury

into the growth plate but be missed on the radiograph. Growth plate injury is very common in the phalanges or the distal radius, so that approximately 70% of all these fractures occur in the upper limb. The distal tibia accounts for just under 10% of the total and the distal femur 1–2%.

A fracture through the growth plate occurs at the zone of hypertrophy: shear produces varying degrees of displacement at the weakest site in the physis where the matrix is minimal and the cells largest [14]. The resistance to shearing or angulation is enhanced by the surrounding tissues, principally the periosteum and the musculoligamentous cuff. Of greater importance is the intrinsic structure of the growth plate including the mammillary (small, cone-shaped) projections that interdigitate with the metaphysis and the overlapping edge (lappet) of the peripheral physis which fits like a cap upon the ossified metaphysis. Surrounding the physis is the groove of Ranvier, which consists of undifferentiated cells capable of increasing the circumference of the growth plate and of anchoring the plate to the perichondrial sheath. A further fibrous band, the perichondrial ring of Lacroix, attaches to the groove of Ranvier [15] and acts as a protective sleeve; this weakens as the skeleton matures. The combination of the Salter–Harris classification and the identification of mechanisms of injury, such as the Lauge-Hansen [16] classification for ankle fractures, allows greater appreciation of the three-dimensional displacement and the best technique for closed reduction [17].

Reduction of paediatric fractures can make use of the more abundant periosteum of childhood which is often intact on the compression side of a long bone fracture. Simple angulation can be corrected with three-point bending with over-correction prevented by the intact periosteum. Translated or off-ended fractures must initially have the deformity exaggerated to relax the intact periosteum on the compression (concave) side of the bone. This will allow careful apposition of the fracture ends before the residual angulation is corrected with bending. Maintenance of the intact periosteum allows effective three-point molding to be applied to support the reduction. This is one of the factors, in combination with the remodeling potential and speed of healing in children, which reduces the need for internal fixation in many paediatric fractures. Management of fractures in a cast should not, however, be considered a simple option. Due vigilance must be given to the technique of cast application to ensure ridges and pressure points are avoided. Care must also be taken to avoid unnecessary restriction of movement of adjacent joints such as the elbow or metacarpal joints by a badly applied forearm cast. Following cast application, the limb should be elevated and observed for signs of evolving neurovascular compromise due to swelling within the cast. Worsening pain, swelling, or pallor of the digits despite elevation mandates splitting of the cast and bandages down to skin without

delay. Loss of fracture reduction should be a secondary concern to preservation of soft tissue and neurovascular integrity. Patients discharged with a recently applied cast should be provided with verbal and written advice regarding the signs of evolving soft tissue problems. The same degree of caution is required after application of a "back-slab" splint as these can be just as restrictive as a complete cast.

Potentially unstable fractures treated in a cast require radiographic surveillance until time and radiological appearance reassure that no redisplacement will occur. Weight bearing should be encouraged as soon as possible after lower limb fracture since there is no evidence that this increases the likelihood of displacement or angulation. Complex regional pain syndrome (algodystrophy) and psychological difficulties occasionally complicate limb fractures in children and satisfactory function is by no means assured where there has been extensive soft tissue injury and vascular impairment.

Overgrowth after a long bone fracture is a well-known problem, particularly in the lower limb. Reynolds [18] considered that this was due to increased vascularity at the time of healing and that the compensatory mechanism thereafter was minimal. The stimulus occurs principally in the first 18 months after trauma, although a further 25% of overgrowth may occur in the subsequent 18 months. Shapiro [19] found that there was a continual, slight overgrowth until maturity, or certainly for the first 4 years after the fracture. There is no clear influence from the dominant limb, and anatomical reduction with internal fixation does not appear to increase the overgrowth. Boys appear to produce a greater degree of overgrowth than girls, although this is an inconstant feature. It is best to allow a 1 cm overlap at the time of femoral fracture splintage or traction in children under 10 years of age in order to accommodate overgrowth of around 1–2 cm. A certain amount of overgrowth will also occur in the ipsilateral uninjured bone of the leg, whether tibia or femur.

Throughout the convalescent period, the parents and child should be kept fully informed of any developments, particularly the concern that further manipulation or even internal fixation may be required. Epiphyseal plate injuries should be reviewed carefully for subsequent growth arrest, which may be either temporary or permanent. The Salter–Harris [20] type V, or sometimes type II, fracture may appear innocent initially, but the effects of growth arrest become increasingly obvious with time.

The problem of growth arrest is dealt with in Chapter 4. Displaced type III and IV fractures should be treated with open reduction and internal fixation, as late as 5 or 7 days after the fracture if necessary. Transepiphyseal fixation with smooth wires is safe and it is advisable to excise the periosteum in order to prevent peripheral bridging. When growth

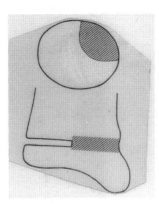

Fig. 1.3 Radiographic projections of a growth tether (osseous bar) will tend to exaggerate the size of the bridge. CT affords a more accurate portrayal of the tether

arrest occurs from a bridging bar of bone, the periphery is involved in 60% of cases (type I), whereas the central (type II) tether occurs in approximately 20% of cases. A combination of patterns (type III) occur in a further 20%.

Surgical procedures to excise the bar must be carried out with precision after preliminary imaging with CT or MRI. At least 50% of the growth plate should be normal, although radiographic projections of the area may exaggerate the bulk of the bar (Fig. 1.3). If the surgery is to be effective, it should be carried out with at least 2 years of potential growth available. Langenskiold and Osterman [21] pointed out that bone shortening maybe treated by a

lengthening procedure or contralateral epiphysiodesis and that angular deformity can be realigned by osteotomy or frame distraction. However, these procedures do not prevent deformation of the joint, which always follows partial closure of the growth plate if the malalignment is allowed to progress (Fig. 1.4a, b).

Baeza Giner and Oliete Sanz [22] studied the use of interposition materials after the excision of an osseous bar. They considered that fat was far more effective than the silastic sheet promoted by Bright [23] and also stated that methylmethacrylate cement [24] caused growth disturbance in its own right.

Indications for Internal Fixation

While the place for internal fixation of fractures in adults is well understood, the indications in children's fractures are more contentious. The existence of multiple variables in childhood fractures such as the age of the child, remodeling potential, and involvement of growth plates has contributed to a lack of large, well-controlled trials. There are, however, broad principles which can guide the decision to treat a fracture surgically.

Three fundamental criteria should be considered:

- the condition of the child
- the age of the child
- the nature of the fracture

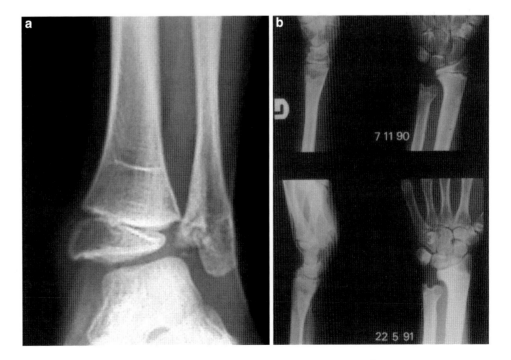

Fig. 1.4 (**a**) Distal fibula physeal arrest has significantly affected ankle alignment. (**b**) Disproportionate growth of the forearm bones after physeal injury (7/11/90) may be checked by distal radial epiphysiodesis (22/5/91) but a later ulnar lengthening is the only means of improving the radio-ulnar relationship

Condition of the Child

The clinical condition influences the decision about internal fixation, either because the injuries pose problems in effective nursing and rehabilitation (e.g., in polytrauma) [25] or severe head injury with behavioral disturbance or because a pre-existing disorder makes conservative management difficult. Some children with skeletal dysplasias, including osteogenesis imperfecta and fibrous dysplasia, cerebral palsy with gross muscle spasm, and mental impairment, are better managed if the fracture is securely fixed at the outset. Pathological fractures of any sort should be considered for operative treatment: This subject is dealt with later in the chapter. Occasionally, social circumstances or concerns about compliance with conservative methods may determine, in part, whether surgical treatment is appropriate.

Age of the Child

Internal fixation is indicated more often in the adolescent, particularly if growth plates are closing when fracture management becomes more akin to the adult situation. In practice, this means that girls older than 12 years and boys older than 14 years may be considered as adults, particularly when dealing with difficult long bone fractures.

Nature of the Fracture

The clinical characteristics of a fracture are determined by

- its site in the bone
- its behavior

Before discussion of the specific anatomical sites at which fixation is often advisable, factors affecting fracture behavior should be considered. Oblique, comminuted, or pathological fractures are usually unstable, and their control may only be achieved with internal fixation. If there is additional bone loss or type III compounding, external fixation with or without subsequent conversion to internal fixation may be required. A fracture may be irreducible by closed means necessitating open reduction which may lower the surgeon's threshold for proceeding to internal fixation. Fracture reduction may be impeded by

- buttonholing through muscle or fascia (lower femoral shaft, proximal humeral shaft, and supracondylar humerus)

- periosteal entrapment (proximal or distal tibia)
- joint incarceration (medial humeral condyle, talus)

Nerve entrapment in the fracture site should also be suspected, particularly in the upper limb at the mid-humeral level, around the elbow, and in the mid-forearm where nerve trunks in relatively anchored sites are close to bare areas of bone between muscle attachments [26]. Muscle contraction may displace fractures producing an unacceptable gap (olecranon and other avulsion injuries) or malalignment (single or double forearm fractures, subtrochanteric femoral fractures).

Primary or delayed internal fixation should therefore be considered for the following reasons, where suitable local expertise allows

- impractical or failed manipulative reduction
- redisplacement of the fracture
- multiple injuries, particularly ipsilateral femoral and tibial fractures (the floating knee)
- significant arterial, neurological, or soft tissue damage where a stable limb facilitates repair
- rare instances of delayed union such as the lateral condyle of the humerus
- displaced intra-articular fractures such as the Tillaux or "triplane" fractures of the distal tibia

Internal Fixation

A wide variety of options exists for the internal fixation of children's fractures. The most common method remains the use of smooth wires. These have the advantages of minimal soft tissue violation and the ability to cross the physis with no noticeable damage. Disadvantages include migration, damage to neurovascular structures, and occasionally infection if used percutaneously. They also have limited stability and require skilful placement to avoid complications and achieve maximal benefit.

Cannulated screw fixation can be very effective for intra-articular fractures such as lateral condylar fractures of the humerus. Plate osteosynthesis remains an option for some long bone fractures. Removal of plates carries a recognized risk of complications as dissection of scarred tissue can lead to neurovascular damage and re-fracture following plate removal. Some choose to leave plates in situ for these reasons but the susceptibility to subsequent fracture at the ends of the plate should be considered.

Elastic nailing of diaphyseal fractures has become increasingly common. For children aged 6–13 years they are the treatment of choice for many types of femoral diaphyseal fractures. They have the advantages of minimally invasive insertion and relatively easy extraction, but their success relies upon good surgical technique and the experience of the user (see Chapters 11 and 12). They may not be appropriate in highly unstable diaphyseal fractures with a likelihood of shortening. This is particularly the case in the treatment of lower limb fracture in older, heavier children (>40 kg). Rigid intramedullary nailing of femoral shaft fractures carries the risk of causing avascular necrosis of the femoral head in skeletally immature children. In adolescents very near skeletal maturity use of a rigid nail with a lateral trochanteric entry point appears to be safe [27].

The use if internal fixation for specific fractures is considered in more detail in later chapters.

Pathological Fractures

Pathological fractures in childhood may occur at any site in the long bones, vertebrae, or pelvis, although they are extremely rare in flat bones. Relatively minor injuries produce the fracture. Characteristically there is no history of convincing trauma, or the incident may be relatively trivial. The child complains of pain, which is usually persistent and sufficient to limit walking if the lower limb is involved. Although the periosteal tube usually prevents significant displacement, the effects of the fracture cannot be ignored.

Internal fixation (see above) will be indicated in specific cases, particularly femoral or tibial fractures. Surgical treatment of fractures associated with conditions of generalized osteopenia such as osteogenesis imperfecta has the advantage of avoiding prolonged immobilization and hence minimizes further loss of bone density from disuse.

Skeletal alterations leading to pathological fracture may be considered as follows:

- generalized
- localized to one limb
- localized to the lesion

The skeletal changes will be either congenital or acquired. The biochemical and biomechanical changes vary, affecting both the composition and the architecture of the bone.

Generalized Conditions

Generalized conditions may be present at birth. Osteogenesis imperfecta [28] is an autosomal recessive disease that may result in multiple fractures at birth and a significantly shortened life span. Birth fractures will be described in Chapter 5 and may be caused by other congenital conditions such as hypophosphatasia and the Silverman syndrome. The child with arthrogryposis who has stiff joints (see Chapter 7 of Children's Neuromuscular Disorders) may also present with a long bone fracture (Fig. 1.5). Proximal femoral pseudarthrosis associated with congenital short femur and pseudarthrosis of the femur may prove confusing·

In later childhood, pathological fractures occur in association with congenital insensitivity to pain (Fig. 1.6), and in osteogenesis imperfecta (Figs. 1.7 and 1.8), whether inherited as autosomal recessive or dominant. Certain of the other skeletal dysplasias such as polyostotic fibrous dysplasia, pycnodysostosis, and osteopetrosis (Fig. 1.9) predispose to pathological or stress fractures, as does osteoporosis of adolescence or the rare juvenile form (Fig. 1.10a, b). The metabolic bone disease associated with end-stage renal or

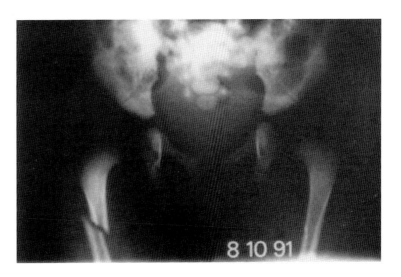

Fig. 1.5 Oblique fracture of the right femoral shaft after the difficult delivery of an arthrogrypotic child

Fig. 1.6 Radiographs of a swollen but painless elbow in a child who was found to be suffering from congenital insensitivity to pain

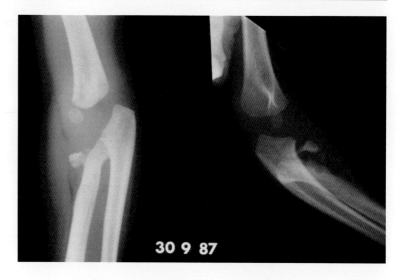

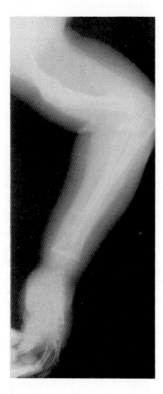

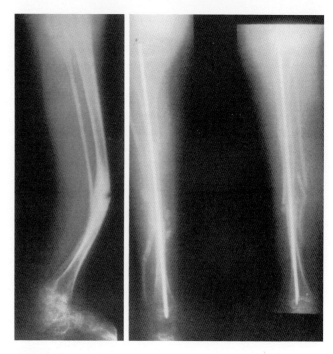

Fig. 1.8 Tibial fracture in osteogenesis imperfecta before and after intramedullary rodding

Fig. 1.7 Upper limb deformity after multiple fracture in osteogenesis imperfecta

hepatic failure is also associated with an increased incidence of fracture, particularly in the convalescent phase after organ transplantation, when steroid therapy and immunosuppression are required. Unusual metabolic conditions such as Bartter's syndrome [29] may be encountered (Fig. 1.11).

Acquired diseases that affect the entire skeleton include leukemias, renal osteodystrophy, hyperparathyroidism, pituitary dysfunction, and infiltrative disorders such as Langerhans' cell histiocytosis. Malnutrition leads to rickets, scurvy, and the wasting diseases (kwashiorkor and marasmus), with concomitant weakening of the skeleton and a predisposition to fracture. These children with their acquired systemic disease are unwell, and the diagnosis must be established if the underlying condition is to be treated effectively. Multiple fractures should also arouse suspicion that the injuries are non-accidental (Chapter 5).

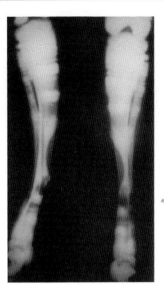

Fig. 1.9 Pathological tibial fractures in a child with osteopetrosis

Single-Limb Involvement

Fractures localized to one limb may be secondary to congenital conditions affecting one or more bones of the limb, such as fibrous dysplasia or Ollier's disease. More commonly, the pathological fracture occurs when disuse osteoporosis results from congenital or acquired conditions. Immobilization or paralytic conditions cause significant bone loss, and rehabilitation must always be graduated and carefully supervised. Myelodysplasia, poliomyelitis, severe cerebral palsy, and arthrogryposis are associated with an increased incidence of fractures, as are chronic osteomyelitis, tuberculosis, septic arthritis, juvenile idiopathic arthritis, post-irradiation osteoporosis, and chemotherapy.

Fractures occur in up to 30% of children with spina bifida [30] and may involve the diaphysis, metaphysis, or growth plate [31]. The diagnosis is often delayed, as the child may not feel pain. Local warmth, erythema, swelling, and progressive deformity should alert the surgeon to the likelihood of pathological fracture. It is easy to confuse the finding with infection. The radiographic appearances may be quite alarming and mimic chronic osteomyelitis [32] or tumor. Congenital insensitivity to pain [33] and post-traumatic neurological loss may also lead to repeated fractures of the weight-bearing bones and to osteolysis. However, blood tests are usually normal and the temptation to take a biopsy of the lesion should be resisted.

The healing of these fractures may be delayed [34], but orthotic support and graduated weight bearing will usually ensure a satisfactory outcome. However, recurrent stress may promote further pathological fracture and a hypertrophic callus response may lead to thickening and deformity around the knee and ankle together with altered growth

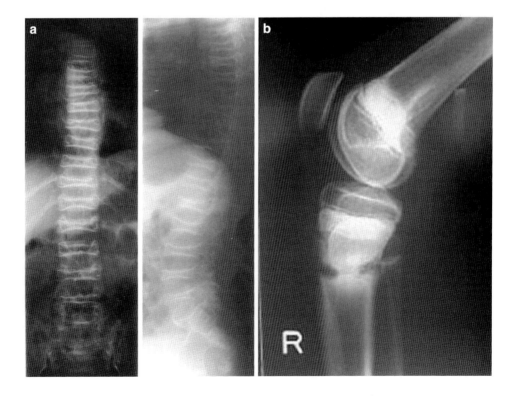

Fig. 1.10 (**a**) Compression fractures of the vertebrae in idiopathic osteoporosis. (**b**) Stress fracture of the proximal tibia in a child with idiopathic osteoporosis. Note the sclerotic metaphyseal bands secondary to bisphosphonate treatment

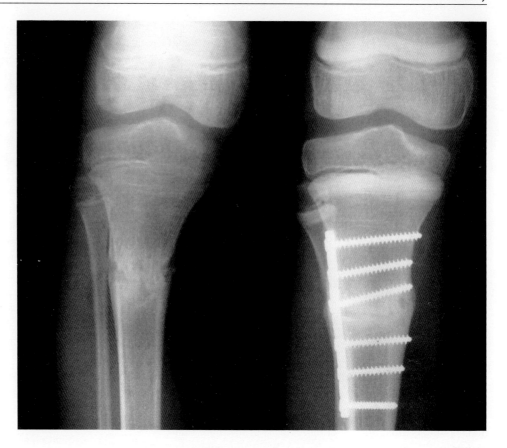

(see Chapter 4). Epiphysiolysis typically produces an initial widening of the growth plate before major slipping occurs. If stress is minimal, the displacement will not progress and the type I epiphyseal fracture [20] will heal slowly.

Monostotic Lesions

Benign cystic conditions of bone are the most common cause of single pathological fracture, which occurs most often in the upper humerus (Fig. 1.12). Although the fracture itself may cause the underlying lesion to heal, needle decompression and injection with steroid or the insertion of bone marrow or cancellous bone graft (Fig. 1.13) may be required before the condition resolves. Splintage may be sufficient in some patients, but a unicameral bone cyst or fibrous dysplasia involving the proximal femur should be fixed in order to prevent varus deformity.

Benign and malignant neoplasms (see Chapter 7 of General Principles of Children's Orthopaedic Disease) and infection (see Chapter 9 in General Principles of Children's Orthopaedic Disease) may cause pathological fracture if cortical destruction exceeds 50% of normal bone strength. A metastatic deposit from nephroblastoma or neuroblastoma (Figs. 1.14 and 1.15) should be included in any

differential diagnosis. Fractures may also occur where the bone has been weakened by the insertion or removal of a screw, pin, or plate, or if blood supply has been impaired by previous trauma, with resultant scarring of the soft tissues.

The typical radiographic appearances include a transverse fracture with little comminution and a relatively indistinct

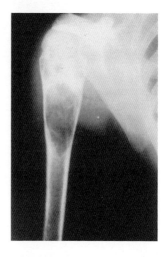

Fig. 1.12 Unicameral cyst of the proximal humerus

Fig. 1.13 A minor pathological fracture through a proximal phalangeal cyst (*left*) was treated by neighbor strapping to the adjacent digit. The cyst healed subsequently (*right*)

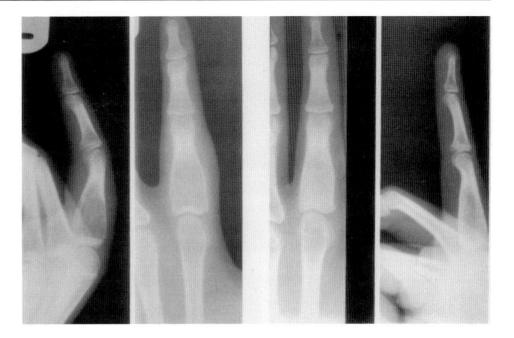

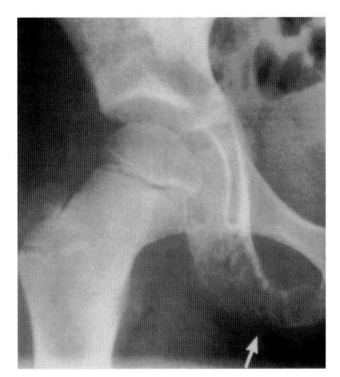

Fig. 1.14 Neuroblastoma metastasized to the inferior pubic ramus

fracture line. Displacement is usually minimal and significant soft tissue wounding is rare. The fracture is usually missed because radiographs are not obtained, although it may be difficult to discern at certain sites, particularly in the spine and ribs. Perthes' disease (see Chapter 6 of Children's Upper and Lower Limb Orthopaedic Disorders) and other examples of osteonecrosis such as osteochondritis of the

femoral condyles, also produce a form of pathological fracture when the ischemic trabeculae are revascularized during the healing process. Finally, congenital pseudarthrosis may sometimes mimic the localized form of pathological fracture, particularly in the absence of cutaneous neurofibromatosis.

Stress Fractures

Stress fractures, while not in themselves "pathological," may also be confusing if a history of repetitive, relatively minor trauma is not sought. In the adolescent, stress fracture of the femoral neck (Fig. 1.16) may occur transversely across the inferior or superior aspects of the neck [35]. The inferior, compression fracture is less likely to displace, but varus deformity resulting from delayed union and persisting symptoms are indications to fix the lesions internally. Stress fractures of the tibia (Fig. 1.17), fibula [36], patella, ulna, and metatarsal have also been described. Chronic epiphyseal and apophyseal changes can be seen in adolescent athletes (Fig. 1.18). Spondylolysis secondary to pathological changes in the pars inter-articularis and spondylolisthesis are discussed in Chapter 1, and chronic stress lesions of the neck, humerus, and ulna are also recognized as rare pathological conditions in childhood.

The tibia usually develops a linear shadow in the proximal metaphysis, and the posteromedial or posterolateral border eventually shows a resorptive fracture line. The midshaft may also thicken anteriorly, similar to the shin splint fracture in the adult. As the fracture line is difficult to see by conventional radiography in the early stages, isotope bone scanning, CT, or MRI are helpful.

Fig. 1.15 CT scan of the pelvic lesion seen in Fig. 1.14

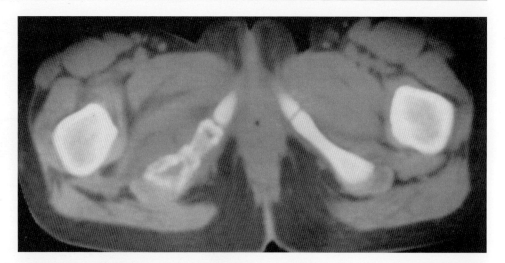

Fig. 1.16 Inferior stress fracture of the right femoral neck

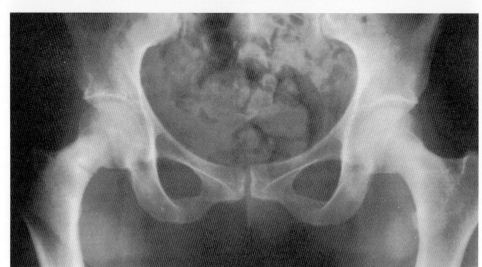

Fig. 1.17 Stress fracture of the proximal tibia in an athletic boy

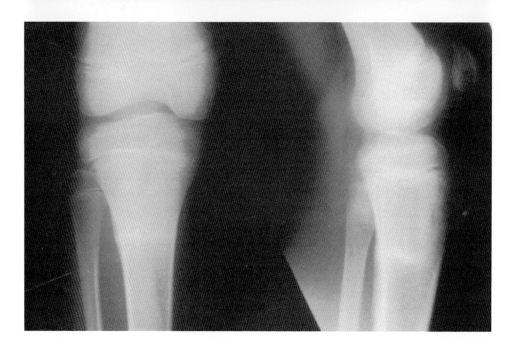

Fig. 1.18 Widened physes and tibial apophyseal fragmentation seen in the knee of a female gymnast

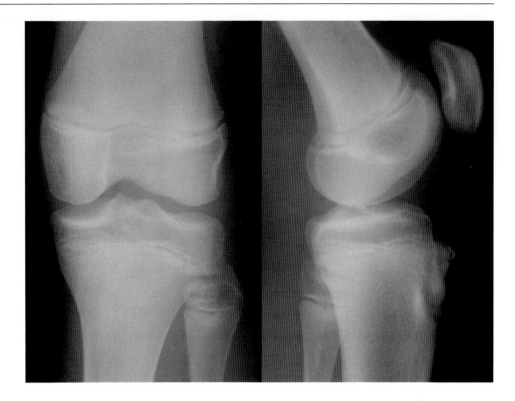

References

1. Jonovska S, Franciskovic T, Kvesic A, et al. Self-esteem in children and adolescents differently treated for locomotor trauma. Coll Anthropol 2007; 31(2): 463–9.
2. Friberg S. Remodeling after distal forearm fractures in children: correction of residual angulation in fractures of the radius. Acta Orthop Scand 1979; 50: 731–9.
3. Poland J. Traumatic separation of the epiphysis. London: Smith Elder; 1898.
4. Konig F. Die spateren Schicksale deform-geheiter Knochenbruche, besonders bei Kindern. Arch Klin Chirurg 1908; 85:187–211.
5. Aitken AP. The end results of the fractured distal radial epiphysis. J Bone Joint Surg 1935:17:302–8.
6. Blount WP. Fracture care in children. Baltimore: Williams & Wilkins; 1954.
7. Pauwels F. Eine Klinische Beobachtung als Beispiel und Beweis fuer funktionelle anpassung des Knochens durch Laengenwachstum. Zeitschrift Orthop 1975; 113:1–5.
8. Crilly RG. Longitudinal overgrowth of chicken radius. J Anat 1972; 112:11–8.
9. Skaggs DL, Friend L, Alman B, et al. The effect of surgical delay on acute infection following 554 open fractures in children. J Bone Joint Surg Am 2005; 87(1):8–12.
10. Ramseier LE, Bhaskar AR, Cole WG, Howard AW. Treatment of open femur fractures in children: comparison between external fixator and intramedullary nailing. J Pediatr Orthop 2007; 27(7):748–50.
11. Gustilo RB, Mendoza RM, William DN. Problems in the management of type III (severe) open fractures: a new classification. J Trauma 1984; 24:742–6.
12. Bae DS, Kadivala RK, Waters PM. Acute compartment syndrome in children: contemporary diagnosis, treatment, and outcome. J Pediatr Orthop 2001; 21(5):680–8.
13. Staudt JM, Smeulders MJC, Van der Horst CM. Normal compartment pressures of the lower leg in children. J Bone Joint Surg Br 2008; 90(2):215–9.
14. Haas SL. Retardation of bone growth by a wire loop. J Bone Joint Surg 1945; 27:25–36.
15. Rang MC. The growth plate and its disorders. Edinburgh: Churchill Livingston; 1969.
16. Lauge-Hansen N. Fractures of the ankle II. Arch Surg 1950; 60:957–985.
17. Dias LS, Giergerich CR. Fractures of the distal tibial epiphysis in adolescence. J Bone Joint Surg 1983; 65-A:438–44.
18. Reynolds DA. Growth changes in long-bones: a study of 126 children. J Bone Joint Surg 1981; 63-B:83–8.
19. Shapiro F. Fractures of the femoral shaft in children: the overgrowth phenomenon. Acta Orthop Scand 1981; 52:649–55.
20. Salter RB, Harris RW. Injuries involving the epiphyseal plate. J Bone Joint Surg 1963; 45-A:587–622.
21. Langenskiold A, Osterman K. Surgical elimination of post-traumatic partial fusion of the growth plate. In: Houghton GR, Thompson GH, eds. Problematic Musculoskeletal Injuries in Children. London: Butterworth; 1983: 14–31.
22. Baeza Giner V, Oliete Sanz V. Profilaxis de los puentes osseous del cartilage de crecimiento. Estudio experimental. Rev Orthop Traumatol 1980; 24: 305–20.
23. Bright RW. Operative correction of partial epiphyseal closure by osseous-bridge resection and silicone rubber implant. J Bone Joint Surg 1974; 56-A:655–64.
24. Mallet J. Les epiphysiodeses patielles traumatique de l'extremite inferieure du tibia chez l'enfant. Rev Chirurg Orthop 1975; 61: 5–16.
25. Loder R. Polytauma in children. Orth Trauma 1987; 1:48–54.
26. Macnicol MF. Roentgenographic evidence of median nerve entrapment in a greenstick fracture. J Bone Joint Surg 1978; 60-A: 998–1000.

27. Kanellopoulos AD, Yiannakopoulos CK, Soucacos PN. Closed, locked intramedullary nailing of pediatric femoral shaft fractures through the tip of the greater trochanter. J Trauma 2006; 60(1):217–22.

28. Sillence DO, Senn A, Danks DM. Genetic heterogeneity in osteogenesis imperfecta. J Med Genetics 1979; 16:101–16.

29. Gill JR. Batter's syndrome. In: Gonick HC, Buckalen VM, eds. Renal Tubular Disorders: Pathophysiology, Diagnosis and Management. New York: Marcel Dekker; 1985.

30. Menelaus MB. The Orthopaedic Management of Spina Bifida Cystica, 2nd ed. Edinburgh: E&S Livingston; 1971:63–65.

31. Parsch K. Origin and treatment of fractures in spina bifida. Eur J Pediatr Surg 1991; 1:298–306.

32. Townsend PF. Cowell HR, Steg NL. Lower extremity fractures simulating infection in myelomeningocele. Clin Orthop Rel Res 1979; 144:256–9.

33. Kuo R, Macnicol MF. Congenital insensitivity to pain: orthopaedic implications. J Pediatr Orthop B 1996; 5:292–5.

34. Wenger DR. Jeffcoat BT, Herring JA. The guarded prognosis of physeal injuries in paraplegic children. J Bone Joint Surg 1980; 62-A:241–6.

35. Devas MB. Stress fractures in children. J Bone Joint Surg 1963; 45-B: 528–41.

36. Griffiths AL. Fatigue fracture of the fibula in childhood. Arch Dis Child 1952; 27:552–7.

Chapter 2

Fracture Epidemiology

Lennart A. Landin

The purpose of fracture epidemiology, as of epidemiology in general, is to identify and describe the etiology of disease in a population, with the ultimate goal of finding methods of prevention. The planning of medical services is also facilitated and made more accurate from epidemiological data. By tradition and out of necessity, the interest of orthopaedic surgeons has focused on diagnosis and therapy but it is also our duty to participate in preventive programs to reduce accidents and to recognize any new hazards that may affect the children in our society. Therefore it is important to have some knowledge of what, why, when, and how the fractures occur in children.

In surveys of paediatric trauma, fractures are found to contribute 10–25% of all injuries in childhood and adolescence [1, 2]. In a series of 23,915 patients seen at four major hospitals for injury-related symptoms in the United States, 17.8% had fractures; thus close to one fifth of children who present to hospitals with injuries have a fracture [3].

Definitions

Incidence is the number of new cases occurring in a defined population during a certain time interval. Thus, the age-specific annual incidence is the risk for an individual or a group of individuals of a certain age of catching a disease or incurring an accident during 1 year.

Prevalence is the total number of persons with a disease or a condition at a certain time in a defined population.

Frequency or *rate* is the percentage of a specific disease or fracture in relation to the total number of cases in a series.

The incidence is dependent upon the accuracy of the sampling procedure and a knowledge of the size of the

L.A. Landin (✉)
Department of Orthopaedics, Malmö University Hospital, Malmö, Sweden

population at risk; minor fractures can escape diagnosis, and severe fractures might be referred to other centers and thus not be recorded. These sources of error should be estimated and non-residents in the population excluded in order to arrive at as precise an incidence as possible. The ultimate goal is to produce reliable data, allowing comparison with other populations, and to detect secular changes. The term incidence is unfortunately often confused with frequency but they are two different entities.

Incidence

The risk of sustaining a fracture, or the incidence, is closely related to age [4]. The incidence of childhood fractures has been calculated in studies from Malmö, Sweden [5, 6], covering 8682 fractures between 1950 and 1979, and 1673 fractures between 1993 and 1994. The risk of fracture increased in children of both sexes up to the age of 11–12 years and then decreased in girls but further increased in boys until the age of 13–14 years (Fig. 2.1). Boys are more commonly represented in all age groups, accounting for 62% of all fractures. From the incidence figures in the Malmö studies, it can be calculated that the cumulative risk of having at least one fracture from birth to the age of 16 years is 42% for boys and 26% for girls, which means that nearly every second boy and every fourth girl will sustain a fracture during the period from birth to the age of 16 years.

The overall annual incidence of fractures was 193 per 10,000, which means that approximately 2% of the children in the population sustain a fracture each year. In a recent study during the year 2000 from Edinburgh, Scotland, the annual incidence of fractures in children was 20 per 1000 and 61% of these fractures occurred in boys [7]. Thus, the incidence and sex distribution are almost identical in these two studies from western Europe.

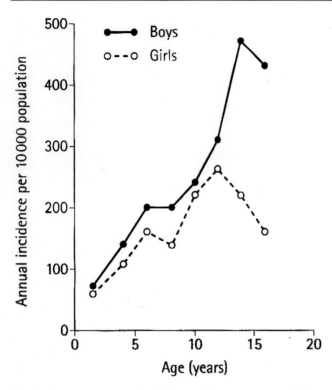

Fig. 2.1 Age- and sex-specific incidence of fractures among children in Malmö, Sweden. (From [5], with permission)

Table 2.1 The frequency of various fracture types

Type	Malmö 1996 (%)	Edinburgh 2000 (%)
Distal forearm	22.7	32.9
Hand (phalanges)	18.9	15.3
Carpus or metacarpal (scaphoid excluded)	8.3	7.6
Clavicle	8.1	7.3
Ankle	5.5	3.5
Tibial shaft	5.0	2.5
Tarsus or metatarsal (talus, os calcis excluded)	4.5	0.3
Foot (phalanges)	3.4	3.0
Forearm shaft	3.4	5.4
Supracondylar region of the humerus	3.3	7.4
Proximal end of the humerus	2.2	1.8
Femoral shaft	1.6	0.7
Vertebrae	1.2	0.35

Frequency

The unique mechanical properties of the growing skeleton, characterized by increased mineralization with age, the function of the periosteum, the presence of the growth plate, physical activity, and psychomotor development, make the fracture pattern in children different from that seen in adults or in the elderly, in whom the loss of bone mass causes the typical patterns of fragility fractures.

In addition, the frequency of the different fracture types, and the incidence of fractures, will be influenced by factors such as age, cultural and environmental factors, and the climate.

The frequencies of the different fracture types in a series of fractures in an urban population in Malmö, Sweden, are shown in Table 2.1 and compared to the Edinburgh data. The most common skeletal injury in children is the fracture of the distal end of the forearm, which contributes to 25% of all fractures, followed by fractures of the hand phalanges and of the carpal and metacarpal regions. Overall, the hand is the most common location of skeletal injury, although many fractures are minor avulsions of little consequence. During the last decade there seems to be an increased incidence and frequency of wrist fractures, accounting for 33% of all fractures in the Edinburgh study. Paediatric fracture patterns are similar in different parts of the world with some exceptions.

In developing countries, road traffic accidents are a much more common cause of fractures as are falls from heights. In a study from Nigeria (1999–2003), femoral shaft fractures accounted for 34%, supracondylar fractures of the humerus 17%, and distal radial factures only 15%. Access to medical services influences the sampling procedure of the data and many minor fractures are likely to be undetected [8].

When the different fracture types are related to age, some patterns can be discerned (Fig. 2.2). The *late peak pattern* is mostly sport and equipment related. The *bimodal pattern* includes an early increase in incidence as a result of low-energy trauma, followed by a late incidence peak, attributable to high- or moderate-energy trauma and again from sport or road accidents. The *decreasing pattern* is typical of skull fractures only. The *rising pattern* is closely related to sports, skateboarding, cycling, and similar activities, which increase with age, particularly in boys. Finally, the *early peak* of the supracondylar fracture of the humerus, mostly caused by falling from a height, and the *irregular pattern* of the tibial shaft are unique for those particular fractures.

Etiology

Environmental Factors

In the Edinburgh study, falls from below bed height accounted for 37%, falls from above bed height 17%, sports-related trauma 12%, and road traffic accidents 6% of all fractures.

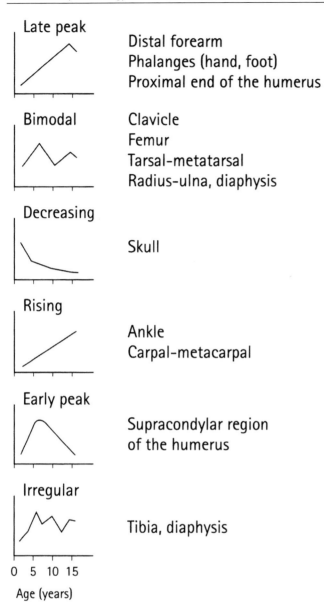

Late peak

Distal forearm
Phalanges (hand, foot)
Proximal end of the humerus

Bimodal

Clavicle
Femur
Tarsal-metatarsal
Radius-ulna, diaphysis

Decreasing

Skull

Rising

Ankle
Carpal-metacarpal

Early peak

Supracondylar region
of the humerus

Irregular

Tibia, diaphysis

0 5 10 15
Age (years)

Fig. 2.2 Patterns of fracture frequency. (From [5], with permission)

New Trends

For several decades, trampolines have been popular as part of playground equipment. In Europe, the recreational use of trampolines has increased during the last 15 years, with an associated increase in the number of children presenting with injuries caused by trampoline use. In a study from Dublin [9], these injuries accounted for 1.5% of the total attendances to the emergency department. Of these, 20% required admission to hospital. Trampolines carry a significant risk of severe orthopaedic injury, the worst being head and spine injuries. In the Irish study, 35% of the patients were on a trampoline with at least one other person. Clear guidelines have been

issued for the safe use of trampolines (Fig. 2.3): only one

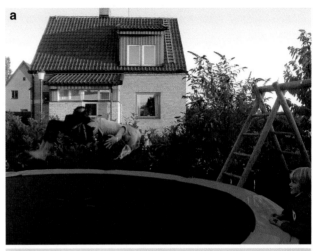

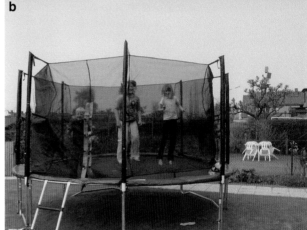

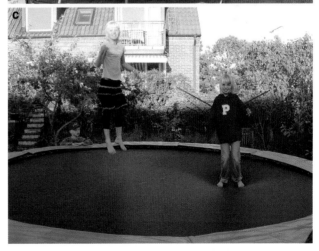

Fig. 2.3 (**a**) Trampoline carry a significant risk of spine and head injuries. (**b**) Trampoline should be fitted with a protective net to prevent falling to the ground and trapping between the trampoline and its frame. (**c**) The smallest child should not be on the trampoline at the same time as the older and heavier ones

person should be on the trampoline at a time and if a number of children are using the trampoline simultaneously, the youngest child is most likely to get hurt. Also, trampolines should be fitted with a peripheral protective net to avoid falls to the ground or trapping between the springs and the frame.

Distal radial fractures have recently been named "the young goalkeeper's fracture." Boyd et al. found that the risk of sustaining a distal radial fracture while goalkeeping was related to the size of the ball [10]. Significantly more injuries were sustained when an adult-sized ball was used instead of a junior ball. One recommendation is also that the goalkeeper should not be younger or smaller than the players in the opposing team.

Other new gadgets are kick boards, motorized scooters, heelies, or street gliders. In a study of injuries caused by using heelies or street gliders, 20% of the injuries happened while using the gliders for the first time and 36% of the injuries occurred while learning how to use them [11]. A similar risk attends the use of skateboards. Most of these injuries are upper extremity fractures and it seems sensible to use wrist protection although the beneficial effects are not scientifically proven.

Endogenous Factors

There has been much debate about whether the etiology of accidents among children reflects not only environmental hazards but also personality traits and social factors. In some investigations, injured children have been found to be impulsive, overactive, impatient, and energetic [12, 13], whereas other studies have shown no personality differences between accident-prone children and control group. It is realistic to accept that "all children are accident-prone sometimes" [14].

Recently, attention deficit hyperactivity disorder (ADHD) has been assessed as a contributing factor to fractures in children. The condition is characterized by permanent and continuous attention deficit with inappropriate hyperactivity or impulsivity, impacting upon all aspects of social life. The conclusions to be drawn from investigations into ADHD and trauma in children are inconsistent, Lam [15] confirming an association while Ford et al. [16] did not.

Children aged 3–6 years and 13–14 years who have sustained one fracture have an increased risk of an additional fracture compared with the overall incidence [5]. Boys are more likely than girls to be "fracture repeaters," which supports the theory that psychological factors are influential.

Children with an evidently fragile skeleton as a result of osteogenesis imperfecta, neurological disorders (such as cerebral palsy, epilepsy, and myelomeningocele), juvenile idiopathic arthritis, and renal osteodystrophy sustain fractures more often than expected, but the scarcity of these conditions makes their contribution to the total number of fractures small. This is in contrast to fractures in the elderly, among whom the majority of patients are osteoporotic or present with associated conditions such as metabolic bone disease, neurological disorders with impaired balance, or rheumatoid arthritis.

In recent decades, the issue of low bone density in children has caused much concern. Landin and Nilsson [17] found that bone mineral content was reduced in 8% of those children who sustained fractures from low-energy trauma, whereas there was no difference in children who sustained their fractures from moderate- or high-energy trauma. In a recent review, Bianchi et al. [18] found an association between reduced bone density and fractures in children. However, there is no distinct pattern of fragility fractures in children as in adults although the quality of the skeleton or the degree of mineralization probably is of importance.

Secular Trends

From 1950 to 1979, the incidence of fractures in children in Malmö, Sweden, almost doubled. The increase was due to a greater number of fractures caused by minor trauma, such as sports-related accidents, whereas high-energy trauma, such as road traffic accidents, decreased over the period. The recorded increase over the years was not explained by improved medical care and access, as the rate of minor avulsions compared with diaphyseal fractures remained constant over the years [5]. A fracture incidence similar to that in Malmö for 1975–1979 was found in children from Nottingham in 1981 [4].

To investigate any further changes in the epidemiology of children's fractures in Malmö, a study covering the years 1993–1994 was performed [6]. The data collection procedure and the organization of the medical facilities were the same as for the study in 1950–1979, allowing an analysis over half a century of paediatric fracture epidemiology in an urban population of western Europe. An overall reduction of 9% in the incidence since 1979 was recorded (Fig. 2.4). It could not be attributed to any single type of skeletal injury or group of fractures. Since the late 1970s, participation in organized sports has increased, whereas unsupervised play has decreased [19]. By 1992, not many more than 50% of 15-year-old Swedish youths engaged in jogging or a corresponding physical effort at least once a week. Although these observations do not constitute direct proof, they can be regarded as circumstantial evidence of the effects of a more sedentary life style upon the risk of fracture. Another explanation could be the effects of safety programs and an increasing awareness of safety among the public in

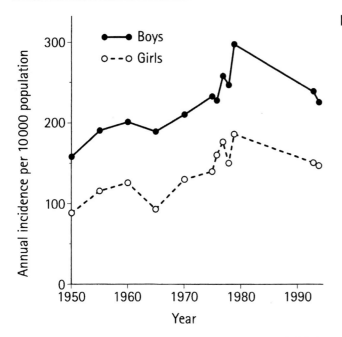

Fig. 2.4 Changes in the incidence of fractures in boys and girls in Malmö, Sweden, from 1950 to 1979 and in the early 1990s

western Europe, exemplified by the use of protective equipment in sports and safety belts in the back seats of cars. The latter, together with the extensive use of specially designed children's seats in cars, have resulted in a threefold reduction in the number of children killed in traffic accidents annually, comparing the periods 1975–1979 and 1993–1994 [20]. However, after 1994 there has been no further reduction; the incidence of lethal traffic accidents in Sweden for individuals 0–17 years in 2007 was per 100,000 annually.

The Future

The incidence of fractures in children seems to mirror the affluence of our society, with sport activities increasing the risk of injury, against a background lifestyle that is more protective and sedentary, governed by video games and computers.

The future will certainly bring new toys, sports, and equipments with associated risks of injuries. Although physical activity is necessary and beneficial for the normal development of the growing child, it is the duty of the paediatric orthopaedic community to act as a whistle blower and initiate preventive measures if fractures and other injuries amass from new devices.

References

1. Sibert JR, Maddocks GB, Brown BM. Childhood accidents—an endemic of epidemic proportions. Arch Dis Child 1981; 56: 225–234.
2. Nathorst Westfelt JAR. Environmental factors in childhood accidents. A prospective study in Göteborg, Sweden. Acta Paediatr Scand Suppl 1982; 53:291.
3. Wilkins KE. The incidence of fractures in children. In: Rockwood CA, Wilkins KE, Beaty JH, eds. Fractures in Children. Philadelphia: Lippincott-Raven; 1996:3–17.
4. Worlock P, Stower M. Fracture patterns in Nottingham children. J Pediatr Orthop 1986; 6:656–660.
5. Landin LA. Fracture patterns in children. Analysis of 8682 fractures with special reference to incidence, etiology and secular changes in a Swedish urban population 1950–1979. Acta Orthop Scand Suppl 1983; 202:1–109.
6. Tiderius CJ, Landin LA, Düppe H. Decreasing incidence in fractures in children. An epidemiological analysis of 1673 fractures in Malmö, Sweden 1993–1994. Acta Orthop Scand 1999; 70: 622–626.
7. Rennie L, Court-Brown CM, Mok JYQ, Beattie TF. The epidemiology of fractures in children. Int J Care Injured 2007; 38:913–922.
8. Nwadinigwe CU, Ihezie CO, Iyidiobi EC. Fractures in children. Niger J Med 2006; Jan-Mar; 15(1):81–84.
9. McDermott C, Quinlan JF, Kelly IP. Trampoline injuries in children. J Bone Joint Surg Br 2006; Jun; 88(6):796–798.
10. Boyd KT, Brownson P, Hunder JB. Distal radial fractures in young goalkeepers: a case for an appropriately sized soccer ball. Br J Sports Med 2001; Dec; 35(6):409–411.
11. Vioreanu M, Sheehan E, Glynn A, et al. Heelys and street gliders injuries: a new type of pediatric injury. Pediatrics 2007; 119(6):e1294–e1298.
12. Mechem Fuller E. Injury prone children. Am J Orthopsychiatr 1948; 18:708–723.
13. Bijur PE, Stewart-Brown S, Bather N. Child behaviour and accidental injury in 11 966 preschool children. Am J Dis Child 1986; 140:487–492.
14. Gustafsson LH. Childhood accidents. Three epidemiological studies on the etiology. Scand J Soc Med 1977; 5–13.
15. Lam LT. Attention deficit disorder and hospitalization due to injury among older adolescents in New South Wales, Australia. J Atten Disord 2002; 6(2):77–82.
16. Ford JD, Racusin R, Daviss WB, et al. Trauma exposure among children with oppositional defiant disorder and attention deficit-hyperactivity disorder. J Consult Clin Psychol 1999; 67(5): 786–789.
17. Landin LA, Nilsson BE. Bone mineral content in children with fractures. Clin Orthop Rel Res 1983; 178:292–296.
18. Bianchi ML. Osteoporosis in children and adolescents. Bone 2007; (41):486–495.
19. Engström LM. Sweden. In: De Knop, P, Engström LM, Skirstad B, Weiss MR, eds. Worldwide Trends in Youth Sport. Champaign IL: Human Kinetics; 1996:231–243.
20. Swedish National Road Administration. Annual Statistics. Borlänge, Sweden: Vägverket Trafikantavdelningen; 1998.

Chapter 3

Polytrauma in Children

Peter P. Schmittenbecher and Cathrin S. Parsch

Introduction

Trauma is still the most common cause of mortality in children, even in countries with the most advanced medical services. Severe head injury carries a high morbidity and mortality, whether isolated or in association with other trauma. However, a fatal outcome is usually the consequence of combinations of injuries. We define "real" polytrauma as two or more system injuries, involved at the same time endangering life as a result of one single or a combination of several injuries. Multiple trauma is always more than the sum of the single injuries; it should be considered as a systemic disease. Orthopaedic injuries account for a high proportion of the damage incurred by the polytraumatized child but are rarely life-threatening in their own right [1].

Scoring Systems

Numerous methods have been developed to classify trauma in adults as well as in children. Anatomical scores, physiological scores, and combined classifications have been promoted. Some authors have concluded that trauma scores especially conceived for use in children fail to show any superiority compared to general trauma scores [2]. Scores seem to be more helpful in the retrospective evaluation of treatment, allowing comparison on a comprehensible basis. They have no crucial influence upon the initial management of patients, although early classification and potential triage on the base of a validated score is still a matter for debate.

The most widely used and accepted scoring systems for children are the modified injury severity score (MISS) and the paediatric trauma score (PTS) [3]. The MISS captures five anatomical body areas with five severity rates (minor to critical), including the Glasgow Coma Scale (GCS) as part of neurological examination (Table 3.1). The score is the sum of the squares of the three most severely injured body areas. More than 25 points indicates an increased risk of permanent disability, and more than 40 points predicts a lethal outcome [4].

The PTS includes six anatomical or physiological components and assigns these severity grades: -1 (major injury), $+1$ (minor injury), or $+2$ (minimal or no injury) (Table 3.2). With more than eight points, no deaths have occurred, with less than zero points the mortality rate was 100%. A linear relationship exists between the PTS and the MISS, but the former can be obtained more easily either at the scene of the accident or in the emergency room and is therefore of use for triage purposes [5].

Epidemiology

It is difficult to obtain reliable data on the incidence of polytrauma in childhood because definitions are vague and the data refer to restricted urban or rural areas. Prospective and obligatory nationwide paediatric trauma registries unfortunately do not exist.

Data from the United States show that 15,000 children (14 years or younger) die each year from accidental injuries, 19 million need some form of medical care, and 100,000 are permanently crippled [6]. The bimodal age distribution has one peak in the first year of life and another during adolescence. The incidence increases with the child's interaction in the outside world (traffic and other accidents) as life moves from the home to out of doors.

In Central Europe, children represent 10–20% of all polytrauma victims. The incidence is estimated to be 360 per 100,000 children. The mortality rate is about 12%. In the German trauma registry, including 17,000 polytrauma cases with an ISS of >16, approximately 6.1% ($n = 1,032$) are children or adolescents under 17 years of age. Every year

P.P. Schmittenbecher (✉)
Department of Pediatric Surgery, Municipal Hospital, Karlsruhe,
Germany

Table 3.1 Modified injury severity score (MISS) [4, 5]

Body area	1 Minor	2 Moderate	3 Severe	4 Life-threatening	5 Critical
Neural	GCS 13–14 Abrasion Contusion	GCS 9–12 Undisplaced facial #	GCS 9–12 Loss of eye Optic nerve avulsion	GCS 5–8 Bone/soft tissue injury with minor destruction	GCS <5 Injuries with airway obstruction
Face and neck	Vitreous or conjunctival hemorrhage Fractured teeth	Laceration of eye Retinal detachment	Displaced facial # Blow-out #		
Chest	Muscle ache Chest wall stiffness	Simple rib # Sternal #	Multiple rib # Hemo-/pneumothorax Diaphragmatic rupture Pulmonary contusion	Open chest wounds Pneumomediastinum Myocardial contusion	Tracheal, aortic, myocardial laceration Hemomediastinum
Abdomen	Muscle ache Seat belt abrasion	Major abdominal wall contusion	Organ contusion Retroperitoneal hematoma Extraperitoneal bladder rupture Thoracic or lumbar spine #	Organ laceration Intraparietal bladder rupture Spine # with paraplegia	Rupture or severe laceration of organs or vessels
Limbs, pelvic girdle	Minor sprains Simple #	Non-displaced # long bones or pelvis	Displaced long bone # Multiple hand/foot # Displaced pelvic # Major nerve/vessel laceration	Multiple closed long bone # Amputations	Multiple open long bone #

= fracture

Table 3. 2 Paediatric Trauma Score (PTS) [5, 6]

	+ 2	+ 1	−1
Size	>20 kg	10–20 kg	<10 kg
Airway	Normal	Maintainable	Unmaintainable
CNS	Normal	Obtunded	Comatose
Systolic blood pressure	>90 mmHg	90–50 mmHg	<50 mmHg
Open wounds	None	Minor	Major, penetrating
Skeletal	None	Closed #	Open or multiple #

33,000 patients suffer from an injury with an injury severity score (ISS) greater than 16; about 2,000 of them are children or adolescents. Males account for 66%, and the incidence mounts with age [7, 8].

Every polytraumatized child should be taken as a warning to reduce accident risks at home, to lobby for the prevention of road traffic accident injuries (e.g., including the use of bicycle helmets), and to ensure that the care of the critically injured child is a clinical priority.

Injuries

Child abuse is the most important cause of polytrauma in the first year of life. In younger children (1–4 years old) falls from a height at home or in the playground are the principal

concern. With increasing age road traffic is the main danger. Motor vehicle collisions with pedestrians and bicyclists are common, yet children are also affected as car passengers if safe seating is not provided or its use enforced.

Principal Patterns of Injuries

Younger children suffer different injury patterns compared to adults. Head injuries and lower limb trauma are more common than thoracic, abdominal, and pelvic injuries (Fig. 3.1). The upper extremity is less often affected. Facial injuries may implicate the cervical spine. First rib and multiple rib fractures are markers for severe trauma and should promote a further search for undetected injuries. Thoracic or lumbar spine trauma suggests additional abdominal injuries. A displaced pelvic fracture warns of other trauma, especially to the abdominal and pelvic cavities.

Falls from a height result in head injuries and a variety of fractures. A typical pattern in a child pedestrian hit by a car comprises head trauma, femoral shaft fracture, and lung contusion. In car passengers 3- or 4-point restraint systems (but not the pelvic restraint belt alone) prevent the characteristic lap-belt injuries: flexion-distraction trauma to the lumbar vertebral column (Chance fracture), disruption of small bowel, and post-traumatic pancreatitis.

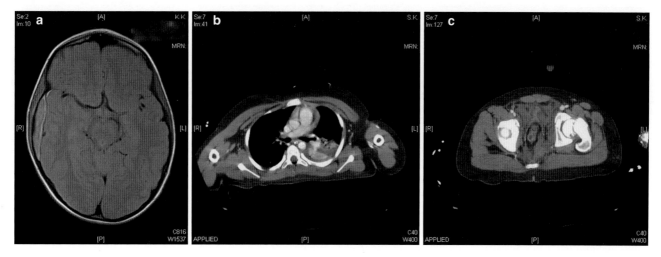

Fig. 3.1 Typical injury pattern in a polytraumatized child with (**a**) an epidural hematoma, (**b**) thoracic (pulmonary) contusion, and (**c**) femoral neck fracture

Generally complications occur in a third of cases, mainly pneumonia and other infections. Mortality is highest with head, thoracic, and abdominal injuries, and the child with an injured cervical spine is at particular risk. Although head and abdominal injuries are often more severe than in adults thoracic trauma carries less hazard than in the adult [9].

A child's neck is short and supports the large head. Due to the flexible spinal column and soft attachments, spinal cord damage and neurological impairment are not necessarily associated with radiological abnormalities. Physiological C2/C3 pseudo-subluxation has to be differentiated radiologically from traumatic spinal injuries.

Specific Physiological and Anatomical Characteristics

Children differ in many physiological and anatomical aspects from adults. The body proportions are quite different, depending on and changing with age. The head occupies a much larger percentage of the body surface and mass compared to adults. The inability of young children to communicate poses an unique challenge in the setting of multisystem trauma.

Airway and Cervical Spine

Recognition and management of airway obstruction and protection of the cervical spine are paramount. The larynx is in a more superior and anterior position, the tongue is larger. The cartilages and soft tissues are softer and more easily compressed. Combined with overall smaller airways especially in the subglottic region, these factors can easily lead to airway obstruction in the setting of an altered conscious state due to head/facial/neck trauma, hypoxia, and hypoperfusion. Post-traumatic mucosal swelling or foreign body obstruction needs additional attention.

Breathing

Hypoventilation is the most common cause of cardiac arrest in children. Compared to adults, the chest wall is more compliant and compressible and the overlying skin and muscles are thin and provide little protection. The elasticity of the cartilaginous ribs allows efficient transmission of a traumatic impact onto the intrathoracic organs. Therefore lung contusions, hemothorax, or diaphragmatic rupture with catastrophic ventilatory and hemodynamic consequences can occur without the rib fractures or clinically obvious external signs of chest trauma. The short, fat neck makes assessment of neck veins and the position of the trachea difficult.

Circulation

Circulatory failure in the setting of multitrauma is mostly due to hypovolemia and blood loss. Other causes are obstruction of venous return (tension pneumothorax and pericardial tamponade) or sympathetic failure (spinal cord injury). In young children in particular the total blood volume is smaller, the stroke volume is fixed, and therefore cardiac output is determined by the heart rate. Tachycardia is usually present but may also be due to pain and anxiety. The age-dependent range for vital signs has to be taken into consideration. Knowledge about age-specific values is important (the normal heart rate for a preschooler is 100–130 beats/min), relative bradycardia for age is a sign of impending cardiac arrest. Other signs of hypoperfusion are decreased central capillary refill, weak pulse pressure, and a decreased level of consciousness due to cerebral hypoperfusion. Blood loss is compensated satisfactorily in the early stages of hemorrhage by vasoconstriction, but decompensation may occur rapidly (talk and die). A decrease in blood pressure is a late sign and resuscitation aims at its prevention.

Abdominal organs are more likely to be injured, as ribs and muscles provide much less protection. Similar to chest injuries, significant internal organ trauma can occur in the absence of obvious external signs. The thoracic spine is seldom affected but lumbar spine (Chance) fractures may occur as part of the lap-belt injury. Chance fractures are usually associated with intra-abdominal injuries. The elasticity of the pelvis prevents severe, unstable disruptions of the ring with severe bleeding.

Disability

The main differences when assessing neurological function relates to preverbal age group. The Paediatric Glasgow Coma Scale has incorporated age-related modifications. Small and seriously ill or injured children are prone to hypoglycemia, which may contribute to the altered conscious state. Sympathetic and adrenal mechanisms as well as relative insulin resistance may cause hyperglycemia, which has been shown to contribute to worse outcomes in the setting of severe head injury.

Exposure/Endocrine

The higher ratio of surface area to volume makes the child vulnerable to hypothermia. Thermal energy loss can occur very quickly and complicate the management of any critically ill or injured paediatric patient.

Furthermore, polytrauma is a systemic disease with a systemic response. Children respond differently to metabolic and physiological stress than adults. The systemic response is reinforced by hypotension, hypovolemia, hypothermia, hypoxemia, pain, and tissue damage and includes a neuroendocrine response (catecholamines, adrenocorticotropic hormones, endorphins, and other local mediators), endotheliopathy, compromised hemostasis, and further dysfunction of temperature regulation. This may be followed by the

release of more mediators, which in turn induce multiple organ failure. But immunological competence and reactive synthesis of cytokines is limited in children. This is the explanation for the low number of systemic inflammatory response syndromes (SIRS) and multiple organ failures (MOF) [8, 10, 11].

Fracture Patterns

Fracture patterns of the limbs in children change with age. In polytrauma minor and incomplete fractures such as greenstick fractures are less frequent because of the higher traumatic energy, but open fractures are more common than usual. The complexity of the soft tissue damage is not a predictor of fracture severity as it is in adults.

Initial Assessment and Management

A structured approach to the seriously injured child enables the timely recognition and management of life-threatening injuries [11–13]. The initial assessment includes

- Primary survey (commences pre-hospital)
- Resuscitation (commences pre-hospital)
- Adjuncts to primary survey (in-hospital)
- Secondary survey
- Emergency treatment and ongoing monitoring
- Definitive care

First Aid, Transport, and Hospital Facilities

The importance of treatment in the pre-hospital phase is well documented since most deaths occur shortly after trauma. As in adults, the most common causes of immediate death are hypoxia, massive hemorrhage, and overwhelming central nervous system (CNS) injury. Scene time should be as short as possible, but during these critical initial minutes, a systematical *primary survey* is vital in identifying life-threatening injuries. The first priority in pre-hospital care is the provision of adequate oxygenation. Multiple attempts at gaining intravenous access should be avoided. Alternative routes such as intraosseous access if available in the pre-hospital environment can be time and life saving.

It is debated whether one should "stay and play" (substitution of volume and intubation) or "load and go" (scoop and run). The decision is influenced by the individual situation.

The child should be managed according to the internationally established principles such as those taught by PALS (Pediatric Advanced Life Support) or APLS (Advanced Pediatric Life Support) courses [11, 13]. Polytraumatized children need a sophisticated and integrated trauma management system specifically focused upon the child. Rapid transport to a dedicated paediatric trauma facility as soon as safely possible is recommended. This means that paediatric intensive care unit (PICU) facilities are required and that experienced paediatric, orthopaedic, and general surgeons are available to assist the emergency team. Paediatric trauma centers have lowered the mortality and morbidity rates, although high costs and geographical restrictions have limited the number of such centers [1, 14, 15]. If this is not possible, then temporary stabilization in a smaller hospital and secondary transfer to a trauma center may be necessary. Communication from the scene or en route enables the receiving facility to mobilize an adequate trauma team, theater, equipment, and blood products as required.

A—Airway

Signs and symptoms of a life-threatening airway or chest injury may be subtle initially, but children can deteriorate rapidly. Supplemental oxygen of around 12 l/min should be supplied. The pharynx is cleared and the neck stabilized in-line with a collar, sandbags, or a tape in neutral position.

Indications for endotracheal intubation are

- inability of the child to protect its airway to prevent aspiration
- inability to ventilate the child with a self-inflating bag-mask system
- altered conscious state or cerebral irritability to protect the airway and prevent further cervical spine injury
- need for controlled ventilation in the context of severe head injury
- ventilatory failure due to severe chest wall and lung injury, e.g., flail chest with paradoxical breathing, pain, exhaustion, and hypoxemia

If intubation is indicated, proper preparation is mandatory. Pre-oxygenation with 100% oxygen, airway opening and clearance (jaw thrust, gentle suction, and airway adjuncts such as an oropharyngeal airway if necessary), as well as preparation of the age/size appropriate instruments and precalculated drugs (rapid sequence induction). Manual in-line stabilization of the cervical spine still provides protection from excessive neck movement.

B—Breathing

After airway maintenance and patency has been secured, acutely life-threatening chest injuries need to be identified and addressed. Asymmetrical chest movement may be difficult to identify in children, as they have small tidal volumes. Signs of increased work of breathing such as accessory muscle use, chest wall retractions, and increasing respiratory rate have to be taken very seriously.

Unilaterally decreased/absent breath sounds, hyperresonant percussion, and tracheal deviation to the opposite side indicate an expanding and tensioning pneumothorax, which has to be decompressed immediately via needle thoracocentesis followed by a large caliber intercostal drain. When aeromedical transfer is undertaken, a Heimlich valve instead of an underwater seal drain is required if tube thoracostomy has been performed.

Unilaterally decreased breath sounds with dull percussion in the context of acute ventilatory and respiratory failure are indicative of a massive hemothorax. The treatment consists of intercostal drainage and fluid resuscitation (including blood transfusion). Thoracotomy may be required.

Flail chest causes paradoxical breathing and is usually accompanied by severe underlying lung contusions. Ventilatory support is generally required.

Pericardial tamponade is rare in blunt trauma. Beck's triad of muffled heart sounds, distended neck veins, and poor perfusion may be difficult to detect in a noisy environment and in the presence of hypovolemia. Immediate pericardiocentesis is followed by emergency thoracotomy. An open pneumothorax (sucking chest wound) is fortunately not a common occurrence. Emergency treatment consists of a bandage taped on three sides followed by a chest drain.

C—Circulation and Hemorrhage Control

Circulatory efficiency depends on the integrity of the "3 Ps"[16]:

- pump (myocardium):
  - Threat: hypoxia and ischemia from hypovolemia
- pipes (integrity of the vascular system)
  - Threat: disruption, organ hypoperfusion due to vasoconstriction
- prime (circulating volume)
  - Threat: hypovolemia due to blood loss or obstruction of venous return (tension pneumothorax and pericardial tamponade)

Indicators of poor perfusion are tachypnea, tachycardia, prolonged capillary refill time, pallor, anxiety, and restlessness. Hypotension occurs late and the child may be obtunded from a combination of intracranial injury as well as cerebral hypoperfusion.

Severe external blood loss is managed by direct manual pressure. Traction splints can also assist in hemorrhage control. Tourniquets should be restricted to exceptional circumstances such as traumatic amputations and are a last resort. Occult blood loss may occur into the thoracic and abdominal cavities, along fractured bones, and into the retroperitoneal space.

Recognizing hemorrhagic shock is essential to ensure good outcomes. Children have an amazing physiological reserve and demonstrate few obvious signs of hypovolemia even when severe volume depletion has occurred. Tachycardia is usually the earliest noticeable response. As mentioned before, knowledge of normal vital signs appropriate for the age of the child is important.

Venous access has to be established before the circulation deteriorates. The insertion of two large bore cannulae is recommended. However, gaining peripheral intravenous access in a child can be difficult, particularly in the presence of shock. After 90 s or 3 failed attempts intraosseous access in a non-fractured extremity should be established. The anterior tibial marrow can usually be cannulated quickly and complications during short-term use are rare. Crystalloids are appropriate for volume substitution (20 ml/kg body weight). If perfusion remains poor after this initial fluid bolus, another bolus of 20 ml/kg is given. If there is still no improvement, O negative blood or group-specific blood, if available (10 ml/kg), must be transfused immediately. Ongoing and repeated assessment of the indicators of adequate perfusion is critical and surgical consultation should be sought early. Although fluid administration should be judicious in the head-injured child, cerebral hypoperfusion due to hypovolemia must be avoided. Once circulatory stability has been achieved, weight-based calculation of maintenance fluids, which should contain glucose, can be ensured whilst monitoring ongoing losses. If the child is moved with an intraosseous needle in place, the flow has to be stopped temporarily before the needle is checked again by aspiration. An unnoticed displacement of the needle tip may cause a compartment syndrome and more importantly prevent further fluid resuscitation, at least temporarily.

D—Disability

CNS injury is the leading cause of death and a presenting GCS of 8 carries a high mortality. However, a rapid assessment of neurological function is performed at the end of the primary survey, because hypoxia, hypoventilation, and hypotension need to be proactively treated to prevent secondary brain damage. Evaluation can include a GCS with age-related modifications, a very quick "AVPU" score (Alert, response to Voice, response to Pain, Unconscious) and a pupillary assessment. A more detailed neurology examination comprises part of the secondary survey.

E—Exposure

Exposure to ambient temperatures and wet weather often render trauma victims hypothermic in the pre-hospital phase.

The patients should be undressed for a full examination and wet garments should be removed immediately as they add to thermal losses. The treating team however has to be aware of the potential heat loss and embarrassment of the child. Warming blankets and devices and (particularly in small children) a heat lamp may be used. If the trauma team receives timely warning about an emergency admission the overall resuscitation room temperature can be raised to prevent further heat loss from the child. Hypothermia, acidosis, and coagulopathy due to hypovolemia comprise the so-called lethal triad [10].

Management of the Multi-injured Child

Adjuncts to the Primary Survey

Full cardiorespiratory monitoring should be established as soon as possible. Radiographic evaluation of the cervical spine, chest, and pelvis is an integral part of the initial assessment of seriously injured children. The interpretation of cervical spine views can be challenging. Depending upon the mechanism of trauma and clinical findings further imaging such as computed tomography (CT) scans may be required. If available a rapid total body projection for the severely injured and unstable child is recommended (Fig. 3.2) [17]. Focused abdominal sonography in trauma (FAST) is gaining more acceptance as a bedside assessment tool in paediatric trauma victims as well. It is mainly useful in the unstable trauma patient where it can reveal free abdominal fluid or pericardial tamponade. In small children ultrasound scans can even identify intracranial injuries.

Bedside glucose (DEFG = Don't Ever Forget Glucose), hemoglobin, and venous blood gas analysis as well as cross/match testing should be obtained as soon as possible.

Aerophagia and manual bag-mask ventilation can cause significant gastric distention. This impedes lung expansion,

Fig. 3.2 Polytrauma CT scan of a pedestrian after collision with a motorcycle. (**a**) An inconspicuous CT, (**b**) pulmonary contusion, (**c**) splenic rupture, (**d**) pelvic fracture, (**e**) open ankle fracture, and (**f**) subcapital humerus fracture

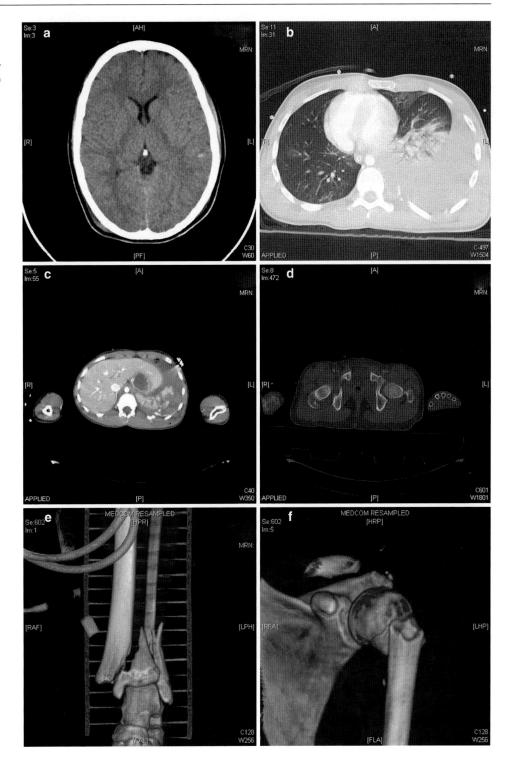

decreases the functional residual capacity, and increases the aspiration risk. Decompression with a nasogastric (in the absence of facial or head trauma) or orogastric catheter can facilitate ventilation. After pelvic fractures and/or ure-thral injuries have been excluded, a bladder catheter can be inserted. This assists in monitoring the adequacy of fluid resuscitative measures.

Secondary Survey

The secondary survey is a detailed evaluation from head to toe and does not begin until the primary survey is completed and resuscitative measures have been established. If at any stage during the secondary survey there is clinical deteri-oration, it is important to reassess ABCDE. Neurological deterioration may have led to airway compromise or a simple pneumothorax may have become a tension pneumothorax; these conditions have to be addressed immediately.

It is very important to document all findings as each system is in a state of flux. Most trauma centers have templates that aid in the assessment and documentation of the examination findings.

The secondary survey of paediatric emergency medicine resource [16] includes SAMPLE history

S Signs and symptoms
A Allergies
M Medications and if immunizations are up to date
P Last medical conditions
L Last meal
E Events before the injuries occurred.

Physical Examination

Head including orifices: Loose teeth and oral bleeding pose an inhalational hazard and can cause airway compromise. As yet unrecognized lacerations, facial injuries including epistaxis and surgical emphysema or ocular damage are important findings. Signs and symptoms of basilar skull fractures, such as hemotympanum, Battle sign, or cerebrospinal fluid otorrhea/rhinorrhea may be detected. Gentle palpation of the head and cranial vault may reveal a boggy scalp hematoma or an underlying skull fracture.

Neck and cervical spine: Without compromising cervical immobilization gentle examination of the neck is important. Midline tenderness and step-offs may indicate underlying bony injury. Increasing swelling, stridor, and surgical emphysema suggest injury to the upper gastrointestinal tract.

Chest: Frequent re-examination of the thorax has to be undertaken so that early signs of deterioration and ventilatory compromise can be detected and reversed. Palpation of the entire bony chest wall as well as looking and listening for symmetry of chest expansion and air entry are mandatory. It has to be remembered that children may sustain major intrathoracic injury with minimal external signs due to the elasticity of the chest wall.

Abdomen: Ecchymosis of the abdominal wall and signs of peritoneal irritation suggest intra-abdominal injuries [18]. About 25% of children with multisystem trauma have a significant abdominal injury. The mortality following blunt abdominal trauma is related to the level of organ involvement: it is less than 20% in isolated solid organ injury and rises to 20% with hollow organ damage. If major vessels are involved, the mortality rises to 50%. External signs may be subtle, and evidence of intra-abdominal blood loss may be masked by the significant ability of children to compensate. Repeated examination (preferably by the same experienced

person) and careful review of ventilatory effort must be ensured.

Pelvis: External palpation will establish tenderness and instability. Perineal bruising or wounds and urethral bleeding are important indicators of major pelvic trauma.

Limbs: The limbs should be examined for deformity, bleeding, and neurovascular dysfunction. Fractured limbs should be temporarily splinted. Frequent re-examination with particular attention to the neurovascular status and skin appearance is important. A high index of suspicion for impending compartment syndrome should mean that this limb-threatening condition is identified early. The effects of extensive soft tissue contusion or lacerations should not be underestimated (Fig. 3.3).

Log roll/examination of the back: Rolling the patient en bloc with the help of several members of the team prevents dangerous movements of the spine. The examiner should look for bruising and open wounds and palpate the spine for abnormal steps, crepitation, and surgical emphysema. In the severely injured child, particularly with lower abdominal/back or pelvic injuries, a rectal examination may be necessary to assess the sphincter tone and the integrity of the rectal wall.

Neurologic examination: During the secondary survey a detailed neurological examination includes motor and sensory examination and reflexes as well as examination of the cranial nerves, orientation, and conscious state. Lumbosacral plexus and sciatic, femoral, or obturator nerve damage may coexist in cases of suspected pelvic fractures.

Adjuncts to the Secondary Survey

The urgency and order of investigations depend on the findings of the primary and secondary surveys. Basic blood tests, plain radiology, and FAST scans can usually be performed whilst resuscitation is being undertaken. Diagnostic peritoneal lavage has been largely abandoned. If emergency surgery is required, some imaging may need to be deferred. Transporting an unstable child out of the resuscitation room into the CT scanner is fraught with danger. This has to be weighed against the need for a definitive diagnosis and anatomical knowledge of injuries present. A team approach involving the surgeon, emergency physician, intensivist, and anesthetist helps to categorize risks and priorities.

Monitoring, Re-evaluation and Analgesia

The severely injured child has to be frequently re-assessed and continuously monitored. Urine output as an indicator of adequate perfusion should be measured by the hourly urine

Fig. 3.3 (a) Soft tissue contusion produced by collision with a bus with (b) a secondary soft tissue defect

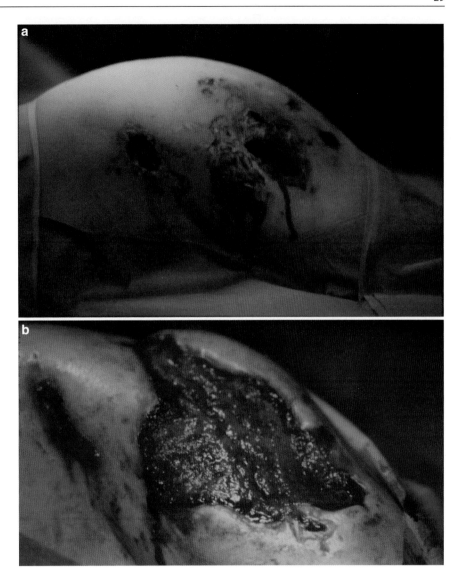

output (provided it is safe to insert a bladder catheter) and 1 ml/kg/h of urine is desirable. Even minor deterioration in vital signs such as relative tachycardia or increase in respiratory rate is significant, as they precede decompensation if not addressed early. Pain relief plays an important part in the management of trauma [19]. Sufficient analgesia and sedation are very important to the child under physical and psychological duress. Intravenous doses of opiates (such as morphine 0.05–0.1 mg/kg using a closely monitored pain protocol) offer effective analgesia without over-sedation and respiratory depression.

Radionuclide scans are useful to identify fractures of different age in cases of non-accidental injury but do not play a role in the emergency setting in a severely injured child. Magnetic resonance (MR) scanning has yet to find a place in the initial evaluation but is of value in later assessment.

Definitive Care

Effective treatment recognizes the control of "threat to life" factors first, followed by the "limitation of disability." So-called damage-control surgery [10] comprises four steps:

1. Control of any significant hemorrhage by compression, ligation, or packs; thorough removal of any contamination; closure of débrided, open wounds; and limb immobilization. These interventions should be completed within 3 h. If emergency operations are necessary, mortality increases in proportion to the time needed for this surgical intervention.

2. Stabilization of the patient in the PICU, including rewarming, correction of coagulopathy, reversal of acidosis, and the monitoring of abdominal and pelvic organ function.
3. Primary phase of definitive surgery within 72 h (for the pelvis, spine, femur, and severe soft tissue injuries)
4. Secondary and tertiary phases of surgery some 10 days after the trauma.

Principles of Treatment

Head Injury

Head injuries are the most common cause of death or long-term disability in children after polytrauma. The severity of head injury correlates with mortality and residual deficits in those who survive, although children often make remarkable recoveries from apparently severe cerebral damage.

A 30° elevation of the head or of the bed, fluid restriction, and slight hyperventilation are the cornerstones of head injury management. Hydration of the patient for volume deficiency or shock has to be achieved carefully in severe brain injury as mentioned previously, yet uncorrected hypovolemia and hypoxemia may also induce secondary brain damage. Diffuse brain edema complicates 30% of cases and if clinical and/or CT signs of head injury or severe edema develop in the unconscious patient intraparenchymatous or intraventricular cerebral pressure monitoring is essential to exclude or confirm significant pressure elevation. The monitoring, fluid management, and ventilation procedures of the severely head-injured child are beyond the scope of this chapter but represent a vital prevention of further brain injury. Early extensive bitemporal craniotomy may be helpful in individual cases if uncontrollable, high cerebral pressure persists. An additional MRI investigation is ensured later to detect brainstem or long-tract injuries if the clinical course is worse than anticipated from the initial CT appearances.

Approximately 10% of children develop post-traumatic seizures after head injuries and prophylactic medication will then be required [20].

The orthopaedic surgeon may be peripheral to many of these therapeutic interventions but still offers an important service in the judicious fixation of fractures, thus minimizing pain and its secondary effects upon intracranial pressure [21].

Spinal Cord Injuries

In multiple trauma a spinal cord injury should be presumed until ruled out. Statistically, 2% of patients have spinal injuries with some element of spinal shock. Cervical spinal cord trauma may occur in typical whiplash injuries and thoracolumbar trauma in lap-belt injuries. A careful examination pays attention to the vertebral column, the surrounding muscle groups, the prevertebral cervical soft tissue, and the peripheral neuromuscular and autonomic function, thus differentiating complete from incomplete lesions. If spinal shock is diagnosed the use of steroids seems to be effective in improving neurologic recovery. Chapter 14 deals with these details. In up to 66% of patients with spinal trauma SCIWORA lesions (spinal cord injury without obvious radiological abnormality) are found with stretching or distraction of the spinal cord in conjunction with the increased elasticity, hypermobility, ligamentous laxity, and immature vascular supply of the spine seen especially in the younger child. Clinical symptoms can develop after a 4-day delay, MR scanning offering an accurate means of assessing the extent of the trauma [1].

Thoracic Injury

The incidence of thoracic injuries is high in polytrauma. Mortality rises to 39% if thoracic trauma is combined with brain and abdominal injury. Although head injury is the main contributor to mortality, morbidity in survivors is influenced by cerebral hypoxia caused by pulmonary deficit.

A first rib fracture or multiple rib fractures are poor prognostic signs because they are indicative of severe trauma. But even without rib fractures, significant intrathoracic injuries may be present. Direct airway injury is rare but is lethal in up to one third of cases. Aortic or diaphragmatic rupture occurs in high-velocity injuries and may be diagnosed from the chest radiograph or the CT scan (Fig. 3.4).

Pulmonary contusion is the most common form of thoracic trauma in paediatric polytrauma and tends to be underestimated on the chest radiograph. If suspected, CT imaging is important because the clinical course of this condition typically deteriorates after a delay, interim extubation and spontaneous breathing worsening matters (Fig. 3.5) [22].

The lung and the kidney are the most significant target organs of secondary damage. Endothelial injury, impaired vascular response, pulmonary vasoconstriction, capillary leak, and interstitial edema are common. In the lung the result is an increase in alveolar capillary permeability, surfactant inactivation, and increased dead space ventilation secondary to intrapulmonary shunts. Respiratory support comprises a limited use of oxygen to prevent toxicity and an adequate positive airway pressure to reduce ventilation/perfusion imbalance.

Fig. 3.4 (**a**) Diaphragmatic rupture with (**b**) peripheral fracture of pelvis

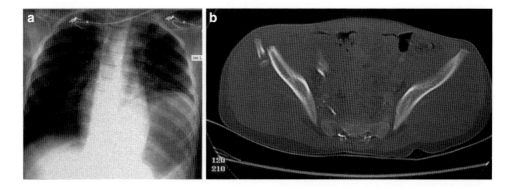

Fig. 3.5 (**a**) Radiograph of the lung with pulmonary contusion compared with (**b**) the CT scan

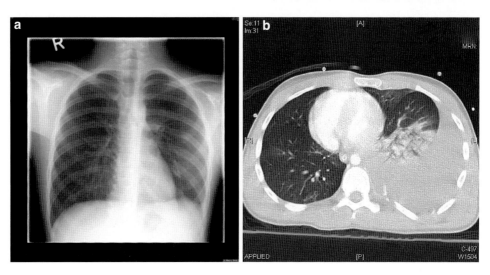

Abdominal Injury

Abdominal injuries occur in one third of polytrauma cases. Trunk ecchymosis is a sign of serious visceral injury, kidney, spleen, and liver being the most often affected. Ultrasound and CT diagnose and classify the injuries accurately. Today most parenchymatous injuries are treated conservatively, but 15% of traumatized kidneys need exploration and reconstruction for renal pelvis laceration or nephrectomy for central disruption [23]. Spleen and liver trauma are stabilized by dealing with the hemorrhage using volume substitution and catecholamine infusions, provided that the blood pressure is stabilized with no more than 40 ml blood transfusion per kilogram body weight per 24 h. With this approach laparotomy is rarely required and the number of splenectomized children is significantly reduced. Even the exploration of an injured liver is seldom indicated, being confined to severe central lacerations or retrohepatic caval tears which make packing essential. The serum transaminase values are a reliable monitor of progress such that abdominal lavage is rarely indicated [24].

Pancreas and gastrointestinal tract are hardly ever involved. Pancreatic contusions are treated like acute pancreatitis. Organ ruptures and lesions of the pancreatic duct are rarely mentioned in case reports. Post-traumatic pseudocysts often resolve spontaneously but large, single cysts may need percutaneous or endoscopic drainage. An enlarging or ruptured cyst, pain, or infection may make an internal surgical drainage via cysto-jejunostomy necessary [25]. Gastrointestinal injuries are found in less than 5% of cases. An obstructing duodenal hematoma is vented by a gastric tube. Perforation of small bowel or colon presents with the signs of peritonitis, and a pneumo-peritoneum is seen on an abdominal radiograph. Bowel rupture should be sutured or resected, followed by anastomosis or enterostomy. This injury is often found in lap-belt injuries and is sometimes identified late since most other parenchymatous organ injuries are now managed without surgery [26].

Orthopaedic Injuries

Skeletal injuries occur in approximately three quarters of polytraumatized children. An emergency intervention is unnecessary except for certain open fractures, vascular damage or a compartment syndrome, and an unstable pelvic or spine fracture. All other cases can be temporarily stabilized, with later elective and definitive management, preferably within 72 h as this improves recovery and rehabilitation [27]. If possible primary definitive fracture care should be achieved at the time of intervention.

The pulmonary benefits of fracture stabilization are not as certain as they are in adults, but longer immobilization undoubtedly increases general complications and an abdominal examination is difficult if a spica cast has been applied. Preliminary fixation with an external fixator during emergency room resuscitation represents a valuable advance in specific cases.

Initially a neurovascular examination is necessary to exclude the necessity of any urgent intervention. In the unconscious child, Doppler studies and possibly compartmental monitoring are appropriate. If vascular repair is necessary, fracture stabilization is essential concurrently or beforehand. In open fractures sterile dressings are applied and tetanus prophylaxis given if the status is unknown.

Femur Fractures

In closed shaft fractures elastic stable intramedullary nailing (ESIN) and external fixator (EF) are the preferred techniques (Figs. 3.6 and 3.7). Both methods are adequate and effective if the surgeon is familiar with the systems. If there is sufficient contact between the main fragments a biomechanically correct insertion of intramedullary elastic nails guarantees correct axis of the limb with enough stability for movement and intensive care and with rapid callus formation. Formation of callus is abundant, particularly in those with head injury. If fractures of the lower limb are at risk of shortening because of a long spiral fracture or a butterfly fragment, end caps can be screwed over the nail ends in the cortical bone and enhance axial stability [28]. When there is bone loss and likely shortening, or a juxta-articular fracture, external monolateral or ring fixators are indicated. In most instances these do not require to be changed before bone union, although occasionally a fixator may be changed to internal fixation later during the recovery period.

Epiphyseal/Metaphyseal Fractures

Metaphyseal fractures are not a major problem but may occasionally merit fixation to aid in nursing care. Epiphyseal fractures are seldom seen with polytrauma. Humeral condylar or ankle fractures are the most common and can be treated with K-wires or screws. In cases of severe, periarticular injury minimal osteosynthesis can be combined with a transarticular, external fixator. Late physeal arrest may

be seen following polytrauma and the details of management are presented in the next chapter.

Open Fractures

Open fractures in children differ from adults' fractures because the degree of soft tissue damage does not predict the complexity of the fracture. Compound fractures can be treated even after a delay of 6–8 h, following the standard principles of copious normal saline irrigation and debridement. Intramedullary fixation with ESIN is effective in first- or second-degree open fractures, reserving external fixation for grade three open fractures, especially degloving injuries of the foot and ankle. Antibiotics are given for 2–3 days or longer depending upon the clinical situation. Wounds are drained and left open if necessary, and in extensive soft tissue loss a temporary coverage is beneficial. Intraoperative cultures correlate poorly with ultimate wound infection and are optional. Soft tissue viability improves with time and facilitates the decision for or against local or free muscle flaps. If an amputation is inevitable, every effort should be made to preserve length and physeal function.

Pelvic Fractures

In pelvic fractures the greater plasticity of bones and the flexibility and elasticity of the sacro-iliac joints and symphysis pubis explain why so much more force is required to produce a fracture than in the adult. These fractures are an indicator of very high-energy injuries (see Chapter 9) and warn about the presence of associated injuries. Retro- and intraperitoneal bleeding from the cancellous bone and disrupted vessels or urogenital trauma are indicated by the presence of a hematoma beneath the inguinal ligament or within the scrotum or by a palpable rectal bony prominence or hematoma. Since pelvic fractures are often stable, they can be managed non-operatively and allow early function. Surgical stabilization is required in horizontal or vertical, unstable pelvic disruption, for rotatory instability or for large, displaced fragments (Fig. 3.8). External fixation reduces bleeding, facilitates transport, and can often be used as the definitive management. Acetabular fractures with displaced fragments and loss of hip joint stability need surgical intervention. Only half of pelvic fractures seen on CT were identified on plain films.

In 9–24% of pelvic fractures genitourinary injury occurs, especially in anterior pubic disruptions. Males are more often affected and urethral disruption is found in the majority of cases (Fig. 3.9). It should be remembered that there is a much bigger symphyseal distance in small children

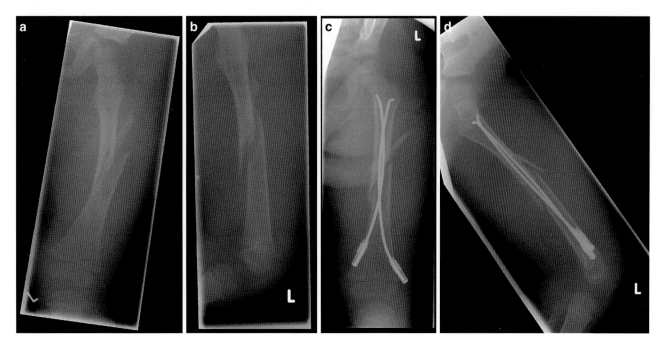

Fig. 3.6 (**a**) and (**b**) Femoral shaft fracture with (**c**) and (**d**) intramedullary nailing using stabilizing end caps

Fig. 3.7 (**a**) Femoral shaft fracture with (**b**) external fixator in place

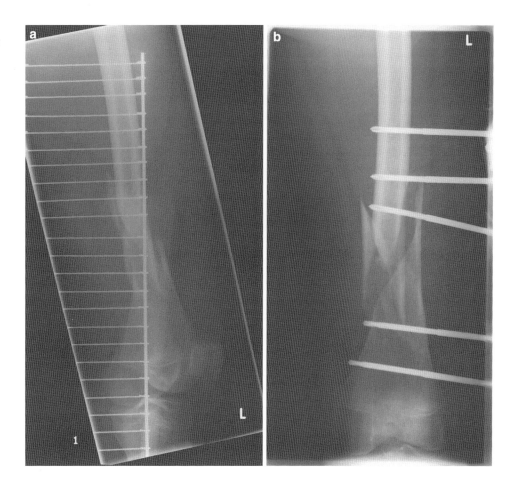

Fig. 3.8 Example of (**a**) and (**b**) unstable pelvic and femoral neck fracture (**c**) and (**d**) after stabilisation with external fixator and femoral neck and sacro-iliac screw fixation

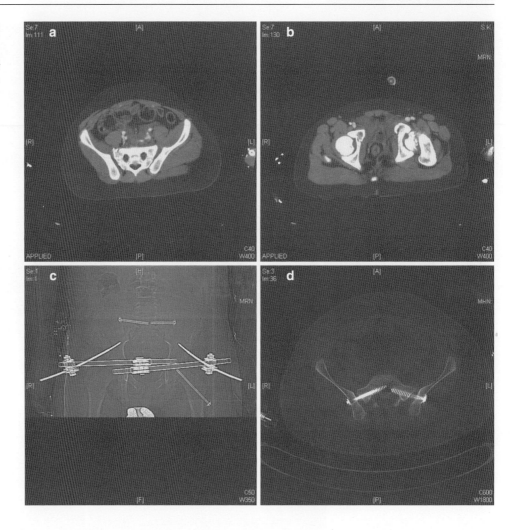

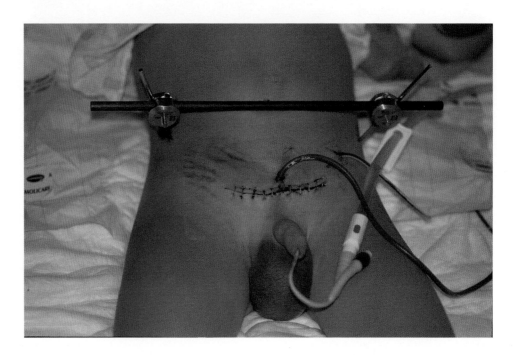

Fig. 3.9 Stabilization of a pelvic fracture with external fixator and reconstruction of urethral disruption

(10–12 mm) compared with adolescents (6 mm) or adults (2–4 mm) [29]. Late diagnosis is common if initial symptoms are not obvious. Care should be taken when inserting a bladder catheter.

Fractures of the Spine

As previously mentioned, the spine is more mobile than in adults and this allows force to be dissipated over a greater number of segments. Hence CT or MR scans show bony contusion and edema over a number of vertebral bodies. Only 1% of paediatric fractures occur in the spine and compression fractures of the thoracic and lumbar segments are more often seen than distraction injuries. Limited spinal fusion is the treatment of choice for the unstable lesion [30].

It is well known that a significant number of skeletal injuries are not identified during the first examination. Therefore repeated and thorough clinical examination is necessary 2–3 days later, augmented by coned radiographs to detect additional skeletal injuries.

A special indication for stabilization is the development of post-traumatic convulsions. Early limb spasticity following severe head injury also makes long bone fracture fixation advisable. In polytrauma, unconventional or atypical surgical interventions may help in the child's recovery, so the surgeon needs to be adaptable.

Psychological Problems

Polytrauma inflicts significant stress upon the child and his family. Emotional shock is followed by denial or depression before recovery takes place. During the first post-traumatic phase psychiatric manifestations may develop and persist throughout a potentially long convalescence.

Outcome, Rehabilitation, and Long-Term Course

The prognosis depends upon the extent of the brain injury [31]. The majority of deaths take place during the first hour and a second peak is found after 48 h. Of those who are not dead on arrival, the mortality rate is approximately 17%.

Long-term disability is seen in 19–28% of all children involved in polytrauma, declining to 12% during the next decade. Nearly half of the relevant functional impairment is the result of brain injury. Five years after the trauma, the signs of focal neurological loss are apparent in one third

of the patients. Neuropsychological and psychosocial problems persist for 6 months in 24% of cases while 42% of brain-injured children following polytrauma exhibit cognitive impairment. The musculoskeletal injuries account for one third of the cases with long-term disability [32–34].

Institutions caring for polytraumatized children need a protocol on how to manage the withdrawal of care for those unfortunate children who cannot be salvaged. Ethical principles must play a part in that very personal and painful decision. The complex problem of organ donation and the dignity of dying require an informed and professional approach.

References

1. Kay RM, Skaggs DL. Pediatric polytrauma management. J Pediatr Orthop 2006; 26:268–277.
2. Ott R, Kramer R, Martus P, et al. Prognostic value of trauma scores in pediatric patients with multiple injuries. J Trauma 2000; 49:729–736.
3. Yian EH, Gullahorn LJ, Loder RT. Scoring of pediatric orthopaedic polytrauma: correlations of different injury scoring systems and prognosis for hospital course. J Pediatr Orthop 2000; 20:203–209.
4. Mayer T, Matlak ME, Johnson DG, et al. The modified injury severity scale in pediatric multiple trauma patients. J Pediatr Surg 1980; 15:719–726.
5. Wilber JH, Thompson GH. The multiply injured child. In: Green NE, Swiontkowski MF, eds. Skeletal Trauma in Children, 3rd ed. Philadelphia: Saunders; 2003.
6. Tepas JJ, Ramenofsky ML, Mollitt DL. The pediatric trauma score as a predictor of injury severity: an objective assessment. J Trauma 1988; 28:425–429.
7. Meier R, Krettek C, Grimme K, et al. The multiply injured child. Clin Orthop Relat Res 2005; 432:127–131.
8. Navascues del Rio JA, Ruiz RMR, Martin JS, et al. First Spanish trauma registry: analysis of 1500 cases. Eur J Pediatr Surg 2000; 10:310–318.
9. Husain B, Kuehne C, Waydhas C, et al. Incidence and prognosis of organ failure in severely injured children and adult patients. Eur J Trauma 2006; 32:548–554.
10. Wetzel RC, Burns RC. Multiple trauma in children: critical care overview. Crit Care Med 2002; 30:468–477.
11. Mackway Jones K, ed. Advanced Pediatric Life Support (APLS), 4th ed. Carlton, Victoria: BMJ Books, Blackwell Publishing Asia; 2005.
12. American College of Surgeons, Committee on Trauma. Advanced Trauma Life Support (ATLS), 7th ed. Chicago: American College of Surgeons; 2002.
13. National Association of Emergency Medical Technicians (U.S.), Pre-Hospital Trauma Life Support Committee; American College of Surgeons Committee on Trauma. PHTLS Prehospital Trauma Life Support, 6th ed. St. Louis MO: Elsevier; 2006.
14. Biaret D, Bingham R, Richmond S, et al. European resuscitation council guidelines for resuscitation, section 6. Pediatric life support. Resuscitation 2005; 67S1:S97–S133.
15. Hall JR, Reyes HM, Meller JF, et al. The outcome for children with blunt trauma is best at a pediatric trauma center. J Pediatr Surg 1996; 31:72–76.
16. American College of Emergency Physicians. The Pediatric Emergency Medicine Resource, revised 4th ed. 2007.
17. Kloppel R, Brock D, Kosling S, et al. Spiral computerized tomography diagnosis of abdominal seat belt injuries in children. Akt Radiol 1997; 7:19–22.

18. Lutz N, Nance ML, Kallan MJ, et al. Incidence and clinical significance of abdominal wall bruising in restrained children involved in motor vehicle crashes. J Pediatr Surg 2004; 39:972–975.

19. O'Donnell J, Ferguson LP, Beattie TF. Use of analgesia in a pediatric accident and emergency department following limb trauma. Eur J Emerg Med 2002; 9:5–8.

20 Morris KP, Forsyth RJ, Parslow RC, et al. UK pediatric traumatic brain injury study group, pediatric intensive care society study-group. Intracranial pressure complicating severe traumatic brain injury in children: monitoring and management. Intensive Care Med 2006; 32:1606–1612.

21. Loder RT, Gullahorn LJ, Yian EH, et al. Factors predictive of immobilization complications in pediatric polytrauma. J Orthop Trauma 2001; 15:338–341.

22. Balci AE, Kazez A, Erern S, et al. Blunt thoracic trauma in children: review of 137 cases. Eur J Cardiothorac Surg 2004; 26:387–392.

23. Delarue A, Merrot T, Fahkro A, et al. Major renal injuries in children: the real incidence of kidney loss. J Pediatr Surg 2002; 37:1446–1450.

24. Stylianos S. Compliance with evidence-based guidelines in children with isolated spleen or liver injury: a prospective study. J Pediatr Surg 2002; 37:453–456.

25. Jobst MA, Canty TG, Lynch FP. Management of pancreatic injury in pediatric blunt abdominal trauma. J Pediatr Surg 1999; 34:818–824.

26. Nance ML, Keller MS, Stafford PW. Predicting hollow visceral injury in the pediatric blunt trauma patient with solid visceral injury. J Pediatr Surg 2000; 35:1300–1303.

27. Magin MN, Erli HJ, Mehlhase K, et al. Multiple trauma in children: pattern of injury—treatment strategy—outcome. Eur J Pediatr Surg 1999; 9:316–324.

28. Dietz H-G, Schmittenbecher P, Slongo T, et al. AO Manual of fracture management. Elastic stable intramedullary nailing (ESIN) in children. Stuttgart: Thieme; 2005.

29. Vitale MG, Kessler MW, Choe JC, et al. Pelvic fractures in children—an exploration of practice and patient outcome. J Pediatr Orthop 2005; 25:581–587.

30. Hasler C, Jeanneret C. Wirbelsäulenverletzungen im Wachstumsalter. Orthopaede 2002; 31:65–73.

31. Rupprecht H, Mechlin A, Ditterich D, et al. Prognostic risk factors in children and adolescents with craniocerebral injuries with multiple trauma. Kongressbd Dtsch Ges Chir 2002; 119: 683–688.

32. Nau T, Ohmann S, Ernst E, et al. Psychopathologic deficits after polytrauma in childhood and adolescence. Wien Med Wochenschr 2003; 153:526–529.

33. Schalamon J, von Bismarck S, Schober PH, et al. Multiple trauma in pediatric patients. Pediatr Surg Int 2003; 19:417–423.

34. van der Sluis CK, Kingma J, Eisma WH, et al. Pediatric polytrauma: short-term and long-term outcomes. J Trauma 1997; 43:501–506.

Chapter 4

Management of Growth Plate Injuries

Franck Accadbled and Bruce K. Foster

Introduction

Treatment of acute growth plate injuries is determined by a prognostic evaluation of the radiographs. The Salter and Harris classification [1] is the most widely used and has been modified by Ogden [2] and more recently by Peterson [3]. The present Ogden classification includes nine major types with subclassifications. For practical purposes the intra-articular fracture line and the degree of initial chondroepiphyseal displacement determine management, as originally proposed by Poland in 1898 [4].

Once there is established growth plate injury, the treatment available is interpositional physiolysis after the method of Langenskiöld [5] with either fat, methyl methacrylate [6], or silastic [7]. Historically, established growth plate deformity with angulation and shortening of the bone has been treated by repeated corrective osteotomy, although transphyseal lengthening [8, 9] and callus distraction [10] can also be considered.

Embryology and Development

Mesenchyme condensations occur in the sixth week of intrauterine life. By the seventh week the condensations become cartilaginous and form anlages that resemble the bones that they will become. The matrix of the cartilage anlage begins to undergo calcification centrally. The periosteal bony cover also starts to be laid down through the process of intramembranous ossification [11].

During the ninth week, vessels invade the newly calcified matrix and begin to remodel the center of the cartilage anlage into bone. The process continues by forming two cartilage plates, one at each end of the bone [11]. The cartilage plates are called the growth plates (physes) and here the process of endochondral ossification responsible for longitudinal bone growth from 9 to 10 weeks' gestational age through to skeletal maturity takes place. The cartilaginous epiphysis at each end of the forming bone also undergoes calcification at a time specific for each bone. It ranges from near birth (e.g., head of the humerus and the proximal tibial epiphysis) to 10–11 years for the lateral epicondyle of the humerus [12].

Endochondral ossification is the process by which bone forms via a cartilaginous intermediary. The growth plate can be divided into at least three zones. The reserve zone is situated on the epiphyseal side of the plate and contains small, spherical cells randomly distributed throughout the zone. It is thought that these cells represent the stem cells which give rise to the chondrocytes in the proliferative zone. In their adjacent proliferative zone, chondrocytes undergo mitosis and are organized into elongated stacks of cells running parallel to the axis of bone growth [13]. Cells in the proliferative zone mature and eventually increase their volume many times in the hypertrophic region. The differentiation and maturation of the chondrocytes together with the associated changes within the matrix surrounding the cells is geared toward producing a microenvironment which encourages mineralization. This culminates in mineralization of the longitudinal septum around the terminal hypertrophic chondrocytes. The mineralized cartilage is then remodeled into true bone in the metaphysis (Fig. 4.1). Much of the process is controlled by growth factors, hormones, and binding proteins, which have the potential to activate or inactivate the growth factors.

Growth hormone has a global effect on physeal function throughout the body, but many growth factors act locally. Of particular interest are parathyroid hormone and parathyroid hormone-related protein (PTHrP) as they can inhibit the maturation of chondrocytes. It is postulated that physeal chondrocytes regulate the local production of PTHrP by secreting a protein (Indian Hedgehog). Indian Hedgehog protein stimulates the chondrocyte to produce PTHrP, which slows the maturation of proliferative chondrocytes to their hypertrophic form [14, 15].

F. Accadbled (✉)
Service de Chirurgie Orthopédique, Hôpital des Enfants, Toulouse, France

Fig. 4.1 A diagrammatic view
of the physis and similar
histological view. Fractures occur
at the weakest level between the
hypertrophic and mineralization
zones

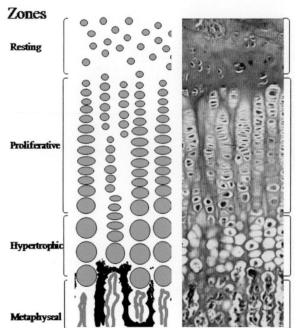

Fig. 4.1 A diagrammatic view of the physis and similar histological view. Fractures occur at the weakest level between the hypertrophic and mineralization zones

Blood Supply

Each growth plate is supplied by the epiphyseal artery from the epiphyseal side and by the main nutrient artery from the metaphyseal side [16].

The epiphyseal artery enters near the capsular insertion point, branches and feeds the numerous capillaries that terminate at the resting side of the physis [17]. While the epiphyseal artery is critical for physeal survival, the metaphyseal vessels are only required for physeal function. Ischemia resulting from damage or destruction of the epiphyseal vessels causes necrosis of the portion of the physis affected [18]. Depending upon the proportion involved, physeal growth can be abolished or differentially slowed leading to angular deformity.

The main nutrient artery enters the diaphysis and branches in the metaphysis to form many small capillaries whose terminal branches invade the matrix between the hypertrophic cells. Interruption to the metaphyseal supply results in a growth plate that can still synthesize cartilage, although mineralization of the cartilage is delayed until the vascular supply has recovered. Upon revascularization the physeal function often returns to normal [18].

Hence, minimizing epiphyseal vasculature injury is important during closed or open fracture reduction and during Langenskiöld procedures. As few pins and screws as possible should be inserted in the epiphysis.

Clinical Condition

Etiology

The junction between hypertrophic and mineralizing cartilage near the metaphysis is biomechanically the weakest point of an adolescent long bone and is therefore the most vulnerable to shearing injury [19]. However, uniform separation does not necessarily occur at that level as the fracture can propagate through different levels of the growth plate. At particular sites, such as the proximal femur, periosteal thinning toward the end of skeletal growth may also predispose to pathological fracture, allowing the upper femoral epiphysis to displace [20]. Hormonal imbalance, irradiation and, in the rat, experimental lathyrism are also contributory factors.

The propagation of the fracture line can occur at different sites through the growth plate, upon which the following classification proposed by Salter and Harris is based [1, 21] (Fig. 4.2).

Type I

There is complete separation of the epiphysis from the metaphysis without any osseous fracture. The growing cells of the physis remain with the epiphysis.

Fig. 4.2 Salter and Harris classification of a physeal fracture. Included here is the important type VI peripheral physeal lesion described by Rang (Reproduced from Rang [21])

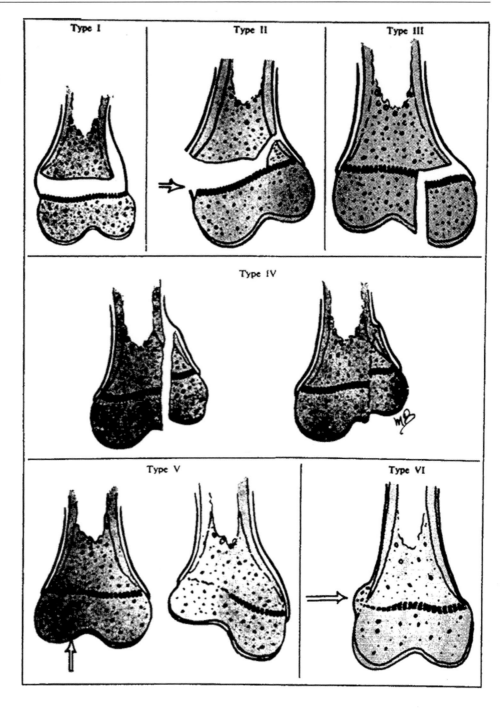

This type of injury occurs in early childhood when the physis is thick. It is also seen in pathological conditions with physeal separation, for example, scurvy, rickets, osteomyelitis, and endocrine imbalance [22]. Wide displacement is uncommon because the periosteal attachment remains intact. Reduction is not difficult, and the prognosis concerning future growth is excellent unless the epiphysis is intra-articular [23], when the blood supply may be damaged and lead to premature closure of the physis (Fig. 4.3).

Type II

The line of separation extends a variable distance along the physis and out through a triangle of metaphyseal bone (the Thurston-Holland sign radiographically). It is the most common type of fracture occurring in 73% of cases [24] (Table 4.1), usually in children over the age of 10 years. The periosteum is torn on the side opposite to the angulation but is intact on the concave side.

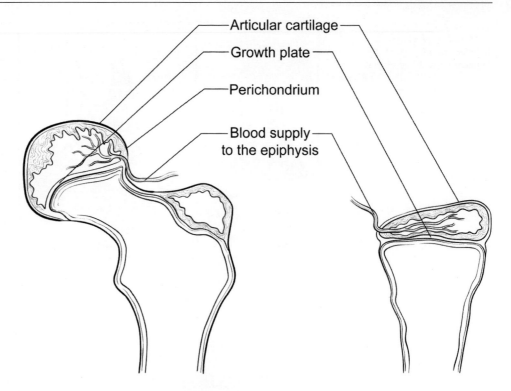

Articular cartilage
Growth plate
Perichondrium
Blood supply to the epiphysis

Table 4.1 Relative frequency of physeal injuries in each location [24]

Physis	No. of injuries (%)
Distal radius	100 (28.3)
Phalanges (fingers)	91 (25.8)
Distal tibia	33 (9.4)
Phalanges (toes)	25 (7.1)
Distal humerus	24 (6.8)
Distal ulna	16 (4.5)
Proximal radius	16 (4.5)
Metacarpals	15 (4.2)
Distal fibula	12 (3.4)
Proximal humerus	7 (2.0)
Metatarsals	5 (1.4)
Proximal tibia	4 (1.1)
Lateral clavicle	3 (0.9)
Proximal ulna	1 (0.3)
Distal femur	1 (0.3)
Total	353 (100.0)

The growing cartilage cells of the physis remain with the epiphysis. The prognosis concerning growth is excellent, provided the circulation to the epiphysis remains intact, which is usually the case.

Type III

The fracture, which is intra-articular, extends from the joint surface to the level of the hypertrophic cells of the physis, and then along the growth plate to its periphery.

The injury is uncommon, but when it occurs it is usually at the upper or lower tibial physis and is caused by intra-articular shearing forces.

Accurate reduction is essential to prevent osseous bar formation across the physis, and to restore a smooth joint surface.

As with type I and II injuries, provided the blood supply to the separated epiphysis is intact, the prognosis is good after accurate reduction.

Type IV

The fracture, which is intra-articular, extends from the joint surface through the epiphysis across the full thickness of the physis and through a portion of the metaphysis, producing complete discontinuity of epiphysis, physis, and metaphysis.

Perfect reduction of a type IV physeal injury is essential if growth and a smooth joint surface are to be restored.

Unless the fracture is undisplaced, open reduction is usually necessary. The physis must be accurately realigned to prevent bony union across the plate with resultant local premature cessation of growth. These fractures occur commonly at the lateral condyle of the humerus, the distal femoral physis, and the distal tibia (Fig. 4.6).

Type V

This relatively rare injury results from a severe crushing force applied through the epiphysis to one area of the physis. It occurs in joints that normally move in one plane only, such as the ankle or knee. At the ankle a severe abduction or adduction force may be applied to the foot, which normally only flexes or extends. The physis is crushed but displacement is unusual, so that the initial radiograph gives little indication of a fracture. The injury may be dismissed as a sprain but where there is localized physeal tenderness, compression of the physis should be suspected. It is postulated but unproven that the risk of premature cessation of growth may be reduced by protection from weight-bearing for 3 weeks.

Rang added the peripheral Ranvier zone injury [21]. This so-called type VI lesion is most commonly associated with a shearing or abrading open injury to the limb such as from a lawn mower or bicycle spoke (Fig. 4.2).

Pathology

Although growth arrest is most common following direct physeal trauma there are many other causes of premature arrest. Idiopathic or pathological avascular necrosis may predispose to growth arrest. For example, patients with Perthes' disease have a 17% incidence [25]. Avascular necrosis secondary to septic arthritis or traumatic hemarthrosis may predispose to growth arrest, as may frostbite, severe burns, irradiation, osteomyelitis, and cannulation injury [26]. The pathology of the growth plate lesion has been defined by experimental work [27]. Bone bridges span the physis with effects similar to the Phemister technique [28] for inducing growth arrest. Fibrous metaplasia may cause the specialized hyaline physeal cartilage to become non-functional fibrocartilage, particularly after avascular necrosis, and this makes treatment of the lesion by interposition methods more difficult.

Incidence

Traumatic and infective physeal injuries do not have a genetic basis. However, Rubin [29] classified the bone dysplasias based upon a dynamic appreciation of their specific structure and function, and observed that heredity did influence both growth and alignment in these conditions.

In reviewing our own experience, the incidence of physeal fractures has been estimated at 17.9% of all fractures that occur in children. They are more common in older children with a peak incidence at 11–12 years of age. Salter-Harris type I displacements made up 8.5% of injuries, type II fractures 73%, type III fractures 6.5%, type IV fractures 12%, and type VI fractures less than 1%. Complication rates are dependent upon the type of fracture, the actual physis involved, and the age of the patient. With accurate open

reduction the complication rate for premature union is in the order of 1–2% [24]. Salter-Harris type IV, V, and VI fractures are much more likely to cause bone bridge formation than types I–III. The distal femur and the proximal tibia account for only 3% of physeal fractures but are responsible for the majority of bone bridges [30]. Rohmiller et al. reported a premature physeal closure rate (PPC) of 39.6% in Salter-Harris II fractures of the distal tibial physis, if there had been insufficient reduction [31]. The site and mechanism of injury therefore can be as important as the degree of severity of the causative violence (Table 4.2).

Table 4.2 The incidence of physeal injuries among 353 children according to the Salter-Harris classification (reproduced from Mizuta et al. [24])

Physis	Salter-Harris type (Figures in parentheses are open fractures)					
	I	II	III	IV	V	Total
Distal radius	7	90 (1)	1	2	0	100
Phalanges (fingers)	7 (1)	74 (2)	8 (1)	2	0	91
Distal tibia	2 (1)	12	8	11	0	33
Phalanges (toes)	1	21 (2)	2	1	0	35
Distal humerus	0	0	0	24	0	24
Distal ulna	2 (1)	12	2	0	0	16
Proximal radius	3	13	0	0	0	16
Metacarpals	0	14	0	1	0	15
Distal fibula	4 (1)	8	0	0	0	12
Proximal humerus	2	5	0	0	0	7
Metatarsals	0	2	2	1	0	5
Proximal tibia	1	2	0	0	1	4
Lateral clavicle	0	1	0	0	0	1
Proximal ulna	0	1	0	0	0	1
Distal femur	0	1	0	0	0	1
Total	30 (4)	257 (5)	23 (1)	42	1	353
Incidence (%)	8.5	73.0	6.5	12	< 1	100

Diagnosis and Differential Diagnosis

Plain anteroposterior and lateral radiographs are the basic investigation in acute growth plate injuries. For complex fractures such as the triplane fracture of the distal tibia, computed tomography (CT) and magnetic resonance imaging (MRI) will give a clearer picture of the fracture pattern. In the patient where there is doubt about the appearance of epiphyseal centers, radiographs of the contralateral side are helpful. For the type V crushing injury there is currently no reliable method of evaluation, although MRI scans may give the earliest indication of growth plate dysfunction [32–35].

Established growth plate injury may be demonstrated by fine-cut CT, which shows the extent of the growth plate arrest. MRI also defines bony bridges but the cortical signal

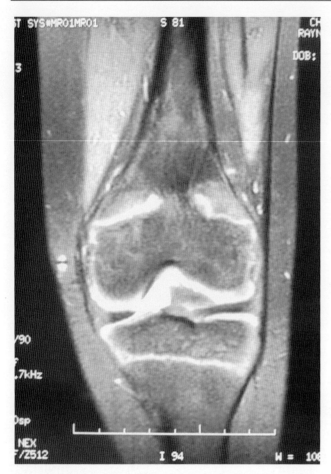

Fig. 4.4 Magnetic resonance image demonstrating central cancellous bone bridging of the distal femoral physis 2 years post injury (Courtesy of Professor Sales de Gauzy)

is similar to that of the cartilage signal and may be confusing (Fig. 4.4). It increases the sensitivity but for bone detail we still prefer CT examination.

The role of isotope bone scanning in determining the extent of growth plate injury is poorly defined. Initial experience suggested that it may be useful to use the bone scan apex view of the distal femur described by Howman Giles et al. [36]. In clinical practice today, however, isotope scanning is probably most helpful in establishing the diagnosis when a fracture is in doubt.

Treatment

Effect of Patient's Age

All patients with the same diagnosis have the same clinical management except for those at the end of their longitudinal growth. If longitudinal growth is almost complete, the need to rescue the physis is diminished. A clinical management flow diagram is presented in Fig. 4.5.

Time of Presentation

Early Presentation

The earlier guidelines of the Salter classification are appropriate. Closed reduction is recommended for all type I and II growth plate fractures. Closed reduction is indicated if the angular displacement is greater than 20° or if there is greater than 20% of epiphyseal displacement. If the child is less than 7 years of age, greater angulations and displacements may safely be accepted. As a working rule, if the limb looks deformed then reduction may be indicated. Follow-up at 1–2 weeks with radiographs is essential to confirm maintenance of reduction. Upper limb splintage is maintained for 4–6 weeks in an above-elbow cast and lower limb splintage for 6–8 weeks in an above-knee cast. Traditionally, weight-bearing is avoided for 2 weeks in the lower limbs.

Should closed reduction fail, judicious open reduction may be indicated. There are certain sites where remodeling is so great that open reduction is rarely indicated. The proximal humeral type II fracture, for example, rarely needs reduction unless there is skin tenting and soft tissue interposition.

Type III and IV injuries usually require open reduction, particularly if the intra-articular displacement is greater than 2 mm. CT, with or without three-dimensional reconstruction, may help to evaluate the displacement. During open reduction, particular care must be taken to prevent damage to the epiphyseal blood supply. Arthroscopically assisted reduction and minimal internal fixation therefore represent an interesting alternative [37]. Minimal internal fixation is best undertaken for 2–3 weeks using Kirschner wires that may or may not traverse the growth plate, or small compression screws placed transversely in the epiphyseal or metaphyseal fragments. Particular care should be taken to avoid damage to the zone of Ranvier. Obliquely placed wires or screws that cross the physis may induce bone bridge formation. Threaded pins or screws that traverse the physis will lead to bone bridge formation [30]. If there is a large metaphyseal fragment, 3.5 mm diameter screw fixation may be all that is required for the metaphyseal fragment. In the distal femur or the distal tibia particularly, intra-epiphyseal screws may provide the most rigid fixation. This is more clearly indicated toward skeletal maturity when avoiding plaster immobilization in addition to internal fixation diminishes joint stiffness (Fig. 4.6).

For comminuted type II, III, IV, and type VI physeal injuries, irrigation and debridement of grossly crushed physeal cartilage and interposition of fat at the time of open reduction and fixation may diminish the risk of bone bridging. The dissection should be restricted in order to reduce potential further damage that may in turn lead to instability

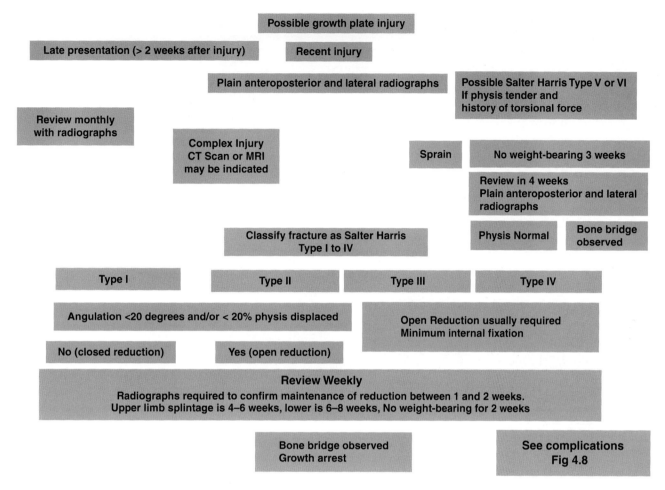

Fig. 4.5 The flow diagram covers the basics of the clinical management of physeal fractures

and deformity. In our experience, early surgical intervention is advisable. Later surgical procedures like osteotomies may need to be repeated until maturity (Fig. 4.7) [38].

Intermediate Presentation

The displaced growth plate fracture seen 2 weeks after injury always poses a management dilemma. Late closed manipulation may further injure the growth plate and it may be prudent to defer treatment and perform a realignment osteotomy later. However, if an open procedure is undertaken, a circumferential metaphyseal-periosteal release may allow gentle repositioning of the grossly displaced epiphysis.

Late Presentation

This is considered under "Salvage Procedures" below.

Complications

Early removal of Kirschner wires after open reduction and internal fixation should prevent pin track infection. For example, following lateral condylar elbow fractures the wires are removed after 2–3 weeks. Biodegradable implants made of synthetic polymers may obviate the need to remove implants but still prove problematical because of local inflammation or their mechanical characteristics. Nevertheless, biodegradable wires have been proved useful in animals and humans [39–46].

With fractures of the distal femoral and proximal tibial physes the risk of associated vascular injury needs to be emphasized. Similarly, compression of the median nerve may occur with markedly displaced distal radial injuries. The site of the growth plate injury is important prognostically. The distal femoral physis, for instance, is most at risk of bone bridge formation and significant premature arrest.

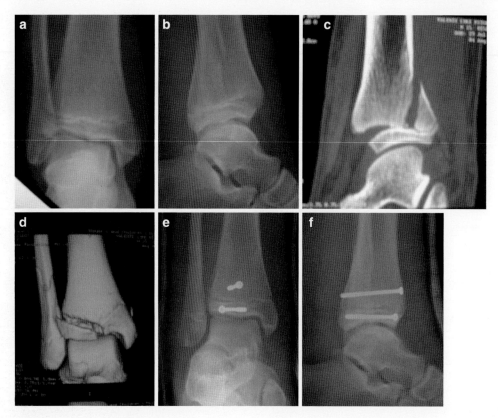

Fig. 4.6 Open reduction of a type IV triplane fracture of distal tibia. Preoperative planning assisted by CT evaluation. Interfragment screw fixation provides intra-epiphyseal and metaphyseal stable fixation. (**a**) Preoperative AP radiograph. (**b**) Preoperative lateral radiograph. (**c**) Preoperative CT scan, sagittal view. (**d**) Preoperative CT scan, 3D reconstruction. (**e**) Postoperative AP radiograph. (**f**) Postoperative lateral radiograph

Salvage Procedures

Once it has been established that bone growth is compromised, techniques used to correct the problem depend upon the physis involved and the age of the patient. Peterson has reviewed the treatment in detail [3, 30, 47]. A clinical flow diagram of the complications is presented in Fig. 4.8.

Possible treatment regimens are described below.

Conservative

If the physeal arrest has occurred near the end of skeletal growth, or in a physis whose contribution to the total length of the limb is minor, the need to excise the bone bridge is small. Limb-length discrepancy of upper limbs is very well tolerated and up to 2.5 cm is acceptable in the lower limbs [30].

Orthoses

Small disparities in lower limb length may be corrected with orthotic support.

Epiphysiodesis (Injured Physis)

Angular deformity in a limb that is almost at the end of skeletal growth may be reduced by destruction of the undamaged portion of the injured physis. This can be performed by placing a staple or screw across the physis. If the limb is already angulated, a corrective wedge osteotomy should be performed (see below).

Epiphysiodesis (Contralateral Physis)

Limb-length discrepancy can be reduced by premature closure of the corresponding physis on the adjacent leg. While this can be achieved by the placement of staples that span the physis on both the lateral and the medial side [48], percutaneous drill epiphysiodesis is now the favored procedure in our center. Screw fixation techniques are sometimes advocated.

Physiolysis

When the bone bridge is likely to lead to unacceptable deformity, the bone bridge itself can be surgically removed.

Fig. 4.7 (**a**) An illustrative case of a 6-year-old boy with a Gustillo compound grade 3 comminuted fracture of the right tibia and fibula sustained in a motor vehicle accident. The wound extended to the medial aspect of the ankle joint which was open. The growth plate of the distal medial tibia was abraded to the bone for 1 cm (*distal arrow*) as in a type VI Rang and Kessel physeal injury. (**b**) Initially the wound was debrided and the fracture stabilized with an external fixator. An acute Langenskiöld procedure was performed for the distal tibial growth plate injury. This included debridement of the exposed peripheral physis with a dental burr and fat interposition. Additionally a rectus abdominal free flap was carried out to cover the skeletal lesion, with splint thickness skin graft to the exposed muscles. The ruptured tibialis anterior tendon was repaired. (**c**) and (**d**) At 3 years 6 months after injury, radiograph confirmed ongoing physeal growth. (**e**) At 4 years and 6 months, CT showed peripheral growth plate repair. At final follow-up 5.5 years later there was no angular deformity of the leg. The distal tibial growth plate was open and the affected limb was 1.5 cm longer than the normal side [38]

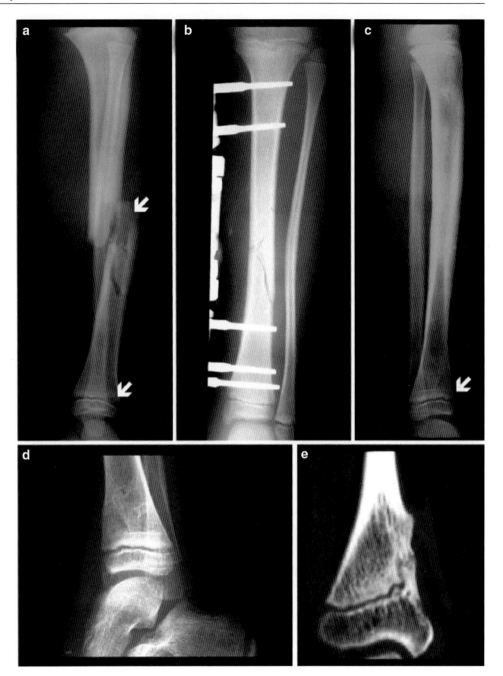

Angular deformity and shortening as a consequence of bone bridge formation can be substantially reduced by timely surgical intervention [24].

The management of growth arrest involves the assessment of angular deformity as well as the extent of the bone bridge. Langenskiöld recommends that, if angulation is greater than 25° at the time of the interpositional physiolysis, a concomitant osteotomy to correct the axis should be undertaken [49]. Interpositional physiolysis may be undertaken within 12 months of normal growth plate closure with an anticipation of correction of length and angulation.

In experimental peripheral growth arrest studies a bridge lesion of up to 17.2% of total physeal area can be treated successfully [50] (Table 4.3). With central lesions as much as 50% of the physeal area may be resected and still allow continued longitudinal growth [6, 49]. Growth arrest is reversed by creating a physiological non-union at the site of the tether so that the remaining physis continues to elongate. This is satisfactory if the critical area of physeal resection is not exceeded and the bone bridge does not reform.

Evaluation of the growth plate lesion is an essential part of the preoperative planning and is best undertaken by CT scans, and more recently by MRI. Physeal mapping using

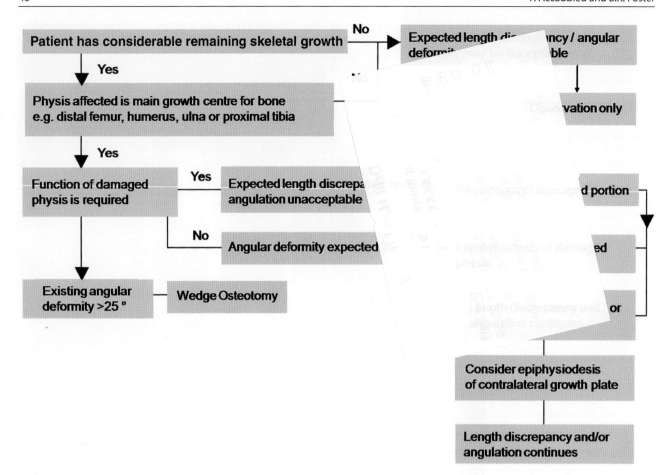

Fig. 4.8 The flow diagram covers the basics of clinical management of the complications that may be expected following physeal trauma

Table 4.3 Reversal by fat interposition in peripheral growth arrest (ovine model) [50]

	CT % area of defect					Reversal success (%)
Reversal groups	Entered	Completed	Sacrifice		Initial	
			3 Months	6 Months		
1 cm^2	20	14	7	7	17.2 ± 2.2	85.7
2 cm^2	15	11	7	4	28.4 ± 6.0	54.5
3 cm^2	10	8	5	3	33.7 ± 7.2	50.0
			Not significant		$P < 0.0001$	

MRI has been demonstrated to be accurate and to offer excellent correlation with intraoperative findings [51–53].

Techniques of Surgery

For a peripheral lesion a longitudinal exposure is made at the anatomical site and, using image intensification, the lesion is identified from the metaphyseal side. After a subperiosteal dissection is made at that point the normal physis and Ranvier zone are identified (Fig. 4.9) using magnification and a dental burr. Damage to the normal growth plate is reduced by irrigation and the bone bridge is then resected completely. Usually fat can be taken from the wound edge to provide the interpositional material. To prevent migration, the fat is sutured to the epiphysis or the perichondrial ring [54]. Bone wax is placed on the bleeding metaphyseal and epiphyseal bone surfaces to reduce the hematoma. Klassen and Peterson [6] have recommended that methyl methacrylate be used as the interpositional material, and Bright [7] has recommended silastic anchored with Kirschner wires. The interpositional material should be anchored to the epiphysis to prevent recurrence [55].

The periosteum is excised at the level of the peripheral lesion to prevent peripheral bone bridge reformation. It is important to place a titanium wire or ball in the epiphysis and metaphysis for subsequent measurement of reconstitution of growth.

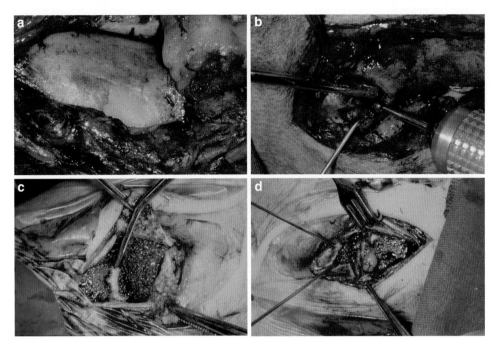

Fig. 4.9 Interpositional physeal surgery. Method of resection of physeal bar. (**a**) Identification of lesion. (**b**) Dental burr and irrigation resection. (**c**) Clear peripheral physeal line. (**d**) Fat transfer and suture to epiphysis

For central lesions the procedure is identical. A larger metaphyseal window is required and visualization of the central lesion is assisted greatly if a powerful light source is used. An arthroscopic cable will sometimes provide a good light source in the small cavity, combined with a dental mirror. Marsh et al. reported on the efficacy of alternating visualization with an arthroscope and burring under fluoroscopy[56].

The bone bridge, whether central or peripheral, may be of ivory cortical or of soft cancellous bone. An additional area that may be difficult to resect is a fibrocartilaginous, nonfunctional growth plate such as occurs after infection. The principal difficulty is to identify the normal ring of growth plate. Resection of the defect should be such that normal growth plate is left circumferentially. Immobilization in a plaster is unnecessary but weight-bearing should be reduced initially in order to prevent impaction fracture into the bone defect.

Limb Lengthening

The procedure of leg lengthening is tedious. It is reserved for the cases in which simple measures have failed. Its role is to regain limb function that is otherwise compromised due to length discrepancy and angular deformity. The procedure, which often takes months to complete, is prone to complications and is outlined in Chapter 4 of Children's Upper and Lower Limb Orthopaedic Disorders.

Conclusions and Future Developments

Physeal injury is common and usually easily diagnosed and treated. Failure to diagnose or to instigate the treatment can lead to significant clinical sequelae. The ability to predict which growth plate injury will lead to premature growth arrest and hence require more aggressive treatment remains a problem. The undiagnosed type V injury may present as a minor injury but may produce extensive arrest, such as a distal radial fracture with subsequent Madelung deformity.

Future developments will also depend upon biological interpositional materials, either physeal cell cultures or the transplantation of physeal cartilage into arrest locations.

Much research has been devoted to finding better ways to repair physeal injury. Most aim to replace the damaged portion with a new tissue.

This has been approached by physeal and chondrocyte transplantation [57–60]. Chondrocyte transplantation has also uncovered a need for better carrier substrates. Three-dimensional biocompatible matrices that enable chondrocyte embedding are slowly being established [61]. Although chondrocyte transplantation has had some success clinically, it still cannot replace large physeal defects. Some of the problems may arise from the inherent polarity of the physis. A physis that is rotated in its vascular bed will continue to produce "metaphyseal bone" on the epiphyseal side [62]. It is hard to envisage how a suspension of cells will determine its own polarity.

Lee et al. demonstrated the feasibility of muscle-based gene therapy and tissue engineering using direct adenovirus-mediated gene transfer to influence reconstruction in injured growth plates [63]. The release of IGF-1 protein after the direct transfer of the IGF-1 gene into the autologous muscle scaffold showed a supportive effect on the restoration of the injured growth plate. The application of mesenchymal stem cells (MSC) also demonstrated some promising results [64, 65].

Further research at the basic level is required. We believe that specific proteins such as growth factors may become key therapeutic tools in the treatment of physeal injuries. Proteins may be able to promote chondrocyte proliferation and migration into defectives zones. Other proteins may be able to inhibit bone bridge formation. However, although some growth factors such as the bone morphogenic proteins (BMPs) are being advocated in the treatment of non-union bone defects, none has yet been shown to aid healing of physeal defects.

References

1. Salter RB, Harris WR. Injuries involving the epiphyseal plate. J Bone Joint Surg [Am] 1963; 45-A: 587–622

2. Ogden JA. Skeletal growth mechanism injury patterns. J Pediatr Orthop.1982; 2:371–377.

3. Peterson H. Physeal injuries and growth arrest. In: Beaty JH, Kasser JR, eds. Rockwood and Wilkins' Fractures in Children. Philadelphia: Lippincott Williams & Wilkins; 2001:91–138.

4. Poland J. Separation of the epiphysis. London: Smith Elder; 1898.

5. Langenskiöld A. An operation for partial closure of an epiphysial plate in children, and its experimental basis. J Bone Joint Surg [Br] 1975; 57-B: 325–330.

6. Klassen RA, Peterson HA. Excision of physeal bars: The Mayo Clinic experience 1968–1978. Orthop Trans 1982; 6:65–75.

7. Bright RW. Operative correction of partial epiphyseal plate closure by osseous-bridge resection and silicone-rubber implant. An experimental study in dogs. J Bone Joint Surg [Am] 1974; 56-A: 655–664.

8. Monticelli G, Spinelli R. Distraction epiphysiolysis as a method of limb lengthening. III. Clinical applications. Clin Orthop Rel Res1981; 154:274–285.

9. De Bastiani G, Aldegheri R, Renzi Brivio L, et al. Chondrodiatasis-controlled symmetrical distraction of the epiphyseal plate. Limb lengthening in children. J Bone Joint Surg [Br] 1986; 68-B: 550–556.

10. Ilizarov GA, Soybelman LM. Some clinical and experimental data concerning bloodless lengthening of the lower extremities. Eksperimental'naya Khirurgiya i Anesteziologiya1969; 14:27–32.

11. Brighton CT. Longitudinal bone growth: the growth plate and its dysfunctions. Instruct Course Lect 1987; 36:3–25.

12. Kaufmann H. Appearance of secondary ossification centers. In: Lentner C, ed. Geigy Scientific Tables, Physical Chemistry, Composition of Blood, Hematology, Somatometric Data. Basle: Ciba-Geigy; 1984:316–318.

13. Johnstone EW, Leane PB, Kolesik P, et al. Spatial arrangement of physeal cartilage chondrocytes and the structure of the primary. J Ortho Sci 2000; 5:302–306.

14. Vortkamp A, Lee K, Lanske, B et al. Regulation of rate of cartilage differentiation by Indian hedgehog and PTH-related protein [see comments]. Science 1996; 273:613–622.

15. Kronenberg HM, Lanske B, Kovacs CS, et al. Functional analysis of the PTH/PTHrP network of ligands and receptors. Recent Prog Horm Res 1998; 53:283–301; discussion 301–303.

16. Harris W. Epiphysial injuries. AAOS Instruct Course Lect1958; 32B: 5.

17. Trueta J, Morgan JD. The vascular contribution to osteogenesis. I. Studies by the injection method. J Bone Joint Surg [Br] 1960; 42:97–109.

18 Trueta O, Amato VP. The vascular contribution to osteogenesis. III. Changes in the growth cartilage caused by experimentally induced ischaemia. J Bone Joint Surg [Br] 1960; 42:571–87.

19. Bright RW, Burstein AH, Elmore SM. Epiphyseal-plate cartilage. A biomechanical and histological analysis of failure modes. J Bone Joint Surg [Am] 1974; 56-A: 688–703.

20. Chung SM. The arterial supply of the developing proximal end of the human femur. J Bone Joint Surg [Am] 1976; 58-A: 961–970.

21. Rang M. The growth plate and its disorders. Edinburgh: Churchill Livingstone; 1969.

22. Salter RB. Textbook of Disorders and Injuries of the Musculoskeletal System. Baltimore: Williams and Wilkins; 1970.

23. Dale GG, Harris WR. Prognosis of epiphyseal separation. An experimental study. J Bone and Joint Surg [Br] 1958; 40:116–122.

24. Mizuta T, Benson W, Foster B, et al. Statistical analysis of the incidence of physeal injuries. J Pediatr Orthop 1987; 7:518–523.

25. Bowen JR, Schreiber FC, Foster BK, et al. Premature femoral neck physeal closure in Perthes' disease. Clin Orthop Rel Res1982; 171:24–29.

26. Macnicol MF, Anagnostopoulos J. Arrest of the growth plate after arterial cannulation in infancy [Br] 2000; 82-B: 172–175.

27. Johnson JTH, Southwick WO. Growth following transepiphyseal bone grafts. An experimental study to explain continued growth following certain fusion operations. J Bone Joint Surg [Am] 1960; 42-A: 1381–1395.

28. Phemister DB. Operative arrestment of longitudinal growth of bones in the treatment of deformities. J Bone Joint Surg [Am] 1933; 15:1–15.

29. Rubin P. Dynamic classification of bone dysplasias. Chicago: Year Book Medical Publishers; 1964.

30. Peterson HA. Partial growth plate arrest and its treatment. J Pediatr Orthop1984; 4:246–258.

31. Rohmiller MT, Gaynor TP, Pawelek J, et al. Salter-Harris I and II fractures of the distal tibia: does mechanism of injury relate to premature physeal closure? J Pediatr Orthop 2006; 26:322–328.

32. Smith BG, Rand F, Jaramillo D, et al. Early MR imaging of lower-extremity physeal fracture-separations: a preliminary report. J Pediatr Orthop 1994; 14:526–533.

33. White PG, Mah JY, Friedman L. Magnetic resonance imaging in acute physeal injuries. Skeletal Radio1994; 23:627–631.

34. Carey J, Spence L, Blickman H, et al. MRI of pediatric growth plate injury: correlation with plain film radiographs and clinical outcome. Skeletal Radiol 1998; 27:250–255.

35. Kamegaya M, Shinohara Y, Kurokawa M, et al. Assessment of stability in children's minimally displaced lateral humeral condyle fracture by magnetic resonance imaging. J Pediatr Orthop 1999; 19:570–572.

36. Howman Giles R, Trochei M, Yeates K, et al. Partial growth plate closure: apex view on bone scan. J Pediatr Orthop 1985; 5: 109–111.

37. Laffosse JM, Cariven P, Accadbled F, et al. Osteosynthesis of a triplane fracture under arthroscopic control in a bilateral case. Foot Ankle Surg 2007; 13:83–90.

38. Foster BK, John B, Hasler C. Free fat interpositional graft in acute physeal injuries. The anticipatory Langenskiöld procedure. J Pediat Orthop 2000; 20:282–285.

39. Bostman O, Vainionpaa S, Hirvensalo E, et al. Biodegradable internal fixation for malleolar fractures. A prospective randomised trial. J Bone Joint Surg Br 1987; 69:615–619.

40. Bostman O, Makela EA, Tormala P, et al. Transphyseal fracture fixation using biodegradable pins. J Bone Joint Surg Br 1989; 71:706–707.

41. Bostman O, Hirvensalo E, Partio E, et al. [Resorbable rods and screws of polyglycolide in stabilizing malleolar fractures. A clinical study of 600 patients]. Unfallchirurg 1992; 95:109–112.

42. Bostman O, Paivarinta U, Partio E, et al. Degradation and tissue replacement of an absorbable polyglycolide screw in the fixation of rabbit femoral osteotomies. J Bone Joint Surg Am 1992; 74: 1021–1031.

43. Makela EA, Bostman O, Kekomaki M, et al. Biodegradable fixation of distal humeral physeal fractures. Clin Orthop Relat Res 1992; 283:237–243.

44. Partio EK, Hirvensalo E, Bostman O, et al. [Absorbable rods and screws: a new method of fixation for fractures of the olecranon]. Int Orthop 1992; 16:250–254.

45. Partio EK, Hirvensalo E, Partio E, et al. Talocrural arthrodesis with absorbable screws, 12 cases followed for 1 year. Acta Orthop Scand 1992; 63:170–172.

46. Hara Y, Tagawa M, Ejima H, et al. Application of oriented poly-L-lactide screws for experimental Salter-Harris type 4 fracture in distal femoral condyle of the dog. J Vet Med Sci 1994; 56:817–822.

47. Peterson H. Treatment of physeal bony bridges by means of bridge resection and interposition of cranioplasty. In: Pablos J, ed. Surgery of the Growth Plate. Madrid: S.A Ediciones Ergon; 1998:299–307.

48. Zuege RC, Kempken TG, Blount WP. Epiphyseal stapling for angular deformity at the knee. J Bone Joint Surg Am 1979; 61:320–329.

49. Langenskiöld A. Surgical treatment of partial closure of the growth plate. J Pediatr Orthop 1981; 1:3–11.

50. Foster B. Epiphyseal plate repair using fat interposition to reverse physeal deformity. An Experimental study. MD, Paediatrics. Adelaide: The University of Adelaide; 1989.

51. Borsa JJ, Peterson HA, Ehman RL. MR imaging of physeal bars. Radiology 1996; 199:683–687.

52. Ecklund K, Jaramillo D. Patterns of premature physeal arrest: MR imaging of 111 children. AJR Am J Roentgenol 2002; 178: 967–972.

53. Sailhan F, Chotel F, Guibal AL, et al. Three-dimensional MR imaging in the assessment of physeal growth arrest. Eur Radiol 2004; 14:1600–1608.

54. Hasler CC, Foster BK. Secondary tethers after physeal bar resection: a common source of failure? Clin Orthop Relat Res 2002; 405:242–249.

55. Jouve JL, Guillaume JM, Frayssinet P, et al. Growth plate behavior after desepiphysiodesis: experimental study in rabbits. J Pediatr Orthop 2003; 23:774–779.

56. Marsh JS, Polzhofer GK. Arthroscopically assisted central physeal bar resection. J Pediatr Orthop 2006; 26:255–259.

57. Foster BK, Hansen AL, Gibson GJ, et al. Reimplantation of growth plate chondrocytes into growth plate defects in sheep. J Orthop Res 1990; 8:555–564.

58. Hansen AL, Foster BK, Gibson GJ, et al. Growth-plate chondrocyte cultures for reimplantation into growth-plate defects in sheep. Characterization of cultures. Clin Orthop Relat Res 1990; 256:286–298.

59. Boyer MI, Danska JS, Nolan L, et al. Microvascular transplantation of physeal allografts. J Bone Joint Surg Br 1995; 77:806–814.

60. Lee EH, Chen F, Chan J, et al. Treatment of growth arrest by transfer of cultured chondrocytes into physeal defects. J Pediatr Orthop 1998; 18:155–160.

61. Sims CD, Butler PE, Casanova R, et al. Injectable cartilage using polyethylene oxide polymer substrates. Plast Reconstr Surg 1996; 98:843–850.

62. Abad V, Uyeda JA, Temple HT, et al. Determinants of spatial polarity in the growth plate. Endocrinology 1999; 140:958–962.

63. Lee CW, Martinek V, Usas A, et al. Muscle-based gene therapy and tissue engineering for treatment of growth plate injuries. J Pediatr Orthop 2002; 22:565–572.

64. Mc Carthy R. Stem cell repair of physeal cartilage. PhD Thesis. Adelaide: The University of Adelaide; 2007.

65. Xian CJ, Foster BK. Repair of injured articular and growth plate cartilage using mesenchymal stem cells and chondrogenic gene therapy. Curr Stem Cell Res Ther 2006; 1:213–229.

Chapter 5

Birth and Non-accidental Injuries

Peter J. Witherow†, Michael K.D. Benson, and Jacqueline Y.Q. Mok

Part I: Birth Injuries

Peter J. Witherow and Michael K.D. Benson

General Considerations

Introduction

The fracture patterns in early infancy differ from those in later childhood and adult life [1]. A knowledge of the infant's bony anatomy helps in understanding how, where, and why fractures occur, particularly in the low-velocity, low-energy skeletal injuries seen in birth trauma and child abuse.

Anatomy

The physis or growth plate tends to be weakest in the hypertrophic and calcifying zones three and four except in infancy: the plane of greatest weakness is then through the ossifying calcified cartilage columns in the metaphysis rather than the deeper layers of the physis. *Fracture separations, therefore, tend to take off a thin shell of juxta-physeal bone.* Peripherally there is a small indentation around the resting and proliferating parts of the growth plate, the groove of Ranvier [2], which contains a zone of increased cellularity. This is associated with bone deposition at the interface between the perichondrium and the physis, producing a thin cuff of bone described by Lacroix as the perichondrial "bone bark" which extends a few millimeters beyond the physis–metaphysis junction, reinforcing it. There is then the zone of bone resorption to establish proper metaphyseal tubulation before laminar bone is deposited at the metaphyseal–diaphyseal junction.

This zone of resorption is associated with a honeycomb-like surface which, particularly in the young infant, represents a point of weakness [3].

The shafts of the neonate's long bones are composed largely of woven bone as Haversian systems are relatively under-developed at birth.

The child's periosteum is thick. It is continuous and densely adherent with the perichondrium of the chondroepiphysis. In the fenestrated area of metaphyseal remodeling, the periosteum is also quite adherent to the fibro-vascular tissue of the inter-trabecular marrow spaces. This stabilizes those metaphyseal fractures which follow the plane of weakness adjacent to the diaphyseal side of the physis so that they tend to heal with minimal subperiosteal new bone. Once this periosteal–bone bond at the metaphysis is broken, however, the loosely applied diaphyseal periosteum can be widely stripped and extensive subperiosteal new bone forms (Fig. 5.1).

Biomechanics

The bone of the neonate and infant is more flexible than that of the older child or adult, although it is not as strong. The load–deformation curve has a long plastic deformation region prior to failure, a characteristic that slows the rate of crack propagation [4]. In the metaphysis and also in the diaphysis of young children, there is relatively little dense lamellar bone and the surface of the propagating crack tends to be irregular rather than relatively smooth. Greater energy is required to drive the fracture line and this restricts its extent.

P.J. Witherow (✉)
Bristol Royal Hospital for Sick Children, Bristol, UK

† It is sad to record the death of Peter J. Witherow, an outstanding children's doctor.

Fig. 5.1 Extensive periosteal reaction following reduction and pin fixation of distal femoral epiphysiolysis in a newborn. This is the post-operative radiograph of the little girl's injury shown in Fig. 5.6

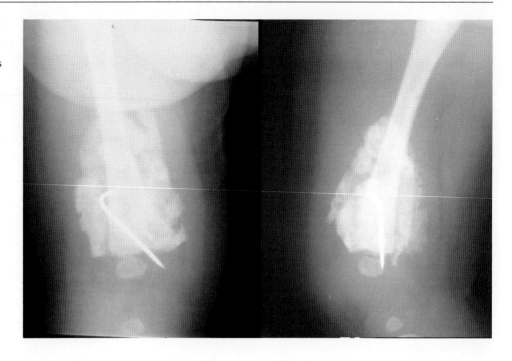

Fracture patterns

Transverse and spiral fractures of the shafts of the long bones occur as in adults and the majority are complete fractures. Incomplete spiral fractures can occur in toddlers, particularly in the tibia, but also sometimes in the femur.

Physeal fracture patterns change as chondroepiphyses mature (only the distal femur regularly has an ossific nucleus at the time of birth): Salter–Harris type I injuries are common in infants; types II, III, and IV become more likely as secondary ossification centers develop and plate undulations enlarge. After the neonatal period, a peripheral fragment which is backed up by the perichondral bone ring of Lacroix frequently remains, with the epiphysis forming the chip or bucket handle appearance seen on radiographs.

Greenstick fractures occur with low-velocity, low-energy injuries when there is failure in tension on one side with plastic deformation or buckling on the other. The woven bone of the young child can also fail largely in compression, which gives rise to metaphyseal torus or buckle fractures usually occurring at the junction between metaphysis and diaphysis, where the transition between the flexible fenestrated and the stiffer cortical bone produces stress concentration.

Healing

The rate of growth of long bones in the first year of life, although decaying, will not be approached again until puberty. Compared with the adult the young child's bones are more vascular and more porous with increased endosteal and periosteal osteogenic potential.

In the neonate, diaphyseal fractures are frequently sticky at a week and stable at three: a toddler may take twice as long to reach the same end points. Remodeling occurs by a combination of periosteal appositional growth and resorptive remodeling together with differential epiphyseal growth.

The potential for remodeling is greatest in the child's first year. Malalignment in the plane of the adjacent joint tends to be best corrected and rotational malalignment worst.

The metaphysis is well vascularized: it is a region of intense bone deposition and remodeling activity and fractures usually heal rapidly.

Birth Injuries

Introduction

Advances in obstetric practice, particularly the more widespread use of Caesarean section to deliver babies presenting by the breech and the better assessment of fetal maturity, have led to a decrease in both the number and the severity of birth injuries. Bruising and lacerations are associated with difficult delivery and episiotomy. Cephalhematoma is common after non-instrumental, vacuum, and forceps deliveries. Brachial plexus palsies may or may not be associated with clavicular fracture. Facial palsy, almost always transient, can follow forceps delivery. Some injuries may be serious and pose difficult problems of diagnosis and treatment.

Incidence

The combined incidence of fractures and brachial plexus injuries has fallen steadily in developed countries: 20 per thousand in the 1930s [5], 7 per thousand in the 1950s [6], and a current level of approximately 2–3 per thousand [7]. The clavicle is most commonly injured followed by the brachial plexus, the humerus, and the femur.

Cervical cord injuries are often present in fatal cases [8], but unidentified fractures of the cervical spine associated with more limited cord or root damage occur more frequently than is appreciated.

The risk of birth injury is increased if manipulation is needed at delivery, if the baby's weight is over 4.5 kg [7], and following breech delivery. Prolonged labor, dystocia,

and prematurity are additional risk factors. Finally fractures are more likely in inflexible children such as those with arthrogryposis (Fig. 5.2).

Etiology

In vertex presentations cervical cord injuries can occur during instrumental rotation of the head from occipito-posterior to anterior in the mid-cavity. They can also result if strong head traction is used to deliver arrested shoulders or, in breech presentations, if heavy traction is used to deliver the after-coming head.

Forceful groin traction during delivery of the extended breech can result in femoral shaft fractures. Humeral fractures may be caused in breech babies when bringing down the arms by hooking a finger into the axilla, particularly when there is shoulder dystocia or the arms are in the nuchal position. Fractures can occur even during Caesarean section delivery [9].

It must be borne in mind that fractures or dislocations may develop in utero. The dislocated hip present at birth may have developed in the later stages of pregnancy, particularly if there were uterine abnormalities, more than one fetus,

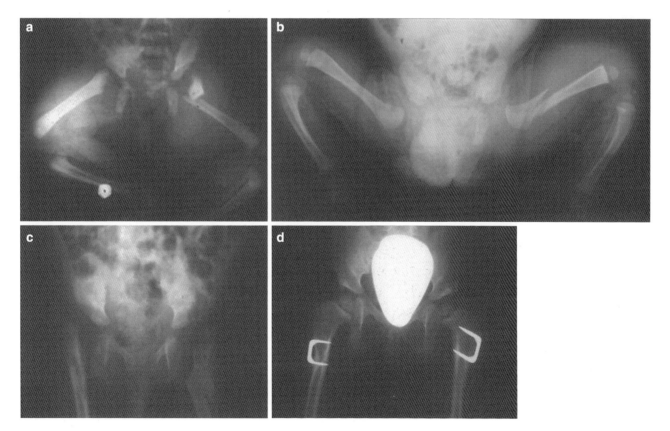

Fig. 5.2 Proximal femoral fracture in a neonate delivered by breech; the child has arthrogryposis and bilateral hip dislocation in addition. (**a**) Initial image. (**b**) In Pavlik harness. (**c**) Fracture union at 5 weeks.

(**d**) Following bilateral open hip reduction and femoral shortening at 12 months or deficient liquor. The dislocated knee similarly reflects a cramped intra-uterine breech position with the knees hyperextended. Fractures may occur antenatally, particularly with severe osteogenesis imperfecta, and are readily diagnosed with routine antenatal ultrasound scans.

Specific Injuries

Clavicle

Clavicular fractures account for 40–50% of all birth injuries. The fracture usually occurs in the mid-third of the bone and is commonly greenstick, although it may be complete and either transverse or oblique. Both shoulder dystocia and large birth weight are risk factors [10]. Most clavicle fractures follow vertex deliveries. Complete fractures of the clavicle are recognized by pseudoparalysis of the ipsilateral arm and pain on handling, but greenstick fractures may not become apparent until 2–3 weeks from the time of delivery when the fracture callus mass becomes obvious.

It is important to exclude an associated brachial plexus palsy because 5% of clavicular fractures are associated with plexus damage [10] and 13% of infants with brachial plexus palsy have a fractured clavicle [11]. It may be difficult to rule out neural injury in the first few days after birth as pain may produce pseudoparalysis or an asymmetrical Moro reflex. The diagnosis normally becomes clear by the end of the first week as the clavicular fracture firms up. Other conditions to be considered in the differential diagnosis of pain around the shoulder are upper humeral osteomyelitis and separation of the proximal humeral epiphysis. Both of these can be differentiated by careful clinical examination.

Congenital pseudarthrosis of the clavicle, although rare, should not be forgotten [12] (see Chapter 22 of Children's Orthopaedics and Fractures). The abnormality may be noted shortly after birth or, more significantly, after discharge home when questions of undiagnosed birth trauma and of possible child abuse may be raised. The pseudarthrosis, unless very rarely bilateral, is on the opposite side to the heart, the bone ends are smooth on radiographs without callus formation, and there is no local tenderness.

Most fractured clavicles need no treatment apart from careful handling. If the fracture is displaced and the baby is in pain, a simple sling made from a crêpe bandage is all that is required.

Shoulder and Proximal Humerus

In the neonate and young infant the junction between the metaphysis and the physis is relatively weak and susceptible to rotational injury. The joint capsule and ligaments fail very infrequently so that dislocations are rare. Most apparent dislocations of the shoulder are therefore fracture separations between the cartilaginous head of the humerus and the metaphysis. This injury produces pain with pseudoparalysis, local swelling, and tenderness around the shoulder. Crepitus is often palpable [13].

The radiographic appearances mimic dislocation because the chondroepiphysis usually lacks an ossific center in the neonate. If there is any uncertainty, ultrasonography (Fig. 5.3) or arthrography can help to confirm that the humeral head is located in the glenoid [14].

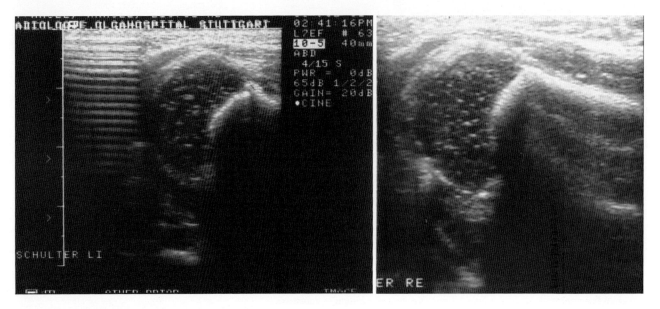

Fig. 5.3 US of proximal humeri in a newborn. Note the left-humeral epiphysiolysis

Treatment is by immobilizing the arm in internal rotation with a sling and swathe. Periosteal new bone appears between the sixth and tenth days and immobilization should be continued for 2–3 weeks.

Distal Humerus and Elbow

Again, dislocation is extremely uncommon, although medial dislocation of the radial head due presumably to forced pronation has been reported [15]. The apparent posterior dislocation is therefore a fracture separation of the distal chondroepiphysis [16, 17] (Fig. 5.4).

Local swelling, tenderness, and possibly crepitus are evident despite the normal relationship between the epicondyles and the tip of the olecranon. The radiologic appearances suggest a posteromedial dislocation but the proximal ends of the radius and ulna lie too close to the lower end of the humerus as the spacer effect of the chondroepiphysis is missing. Ultrasound or arthrography will confirm the diagnosis.

Treatment should be by re-alignment with splintage of the elbow in a sling and swathe or a posterior slab for 2–3 weeks. Recovery is usually very satisfactory.

Humeral and Femoral Shaft Fractures

Most fractures are mid-third, transverse, and complete (Fig. 5.5). For the humerus, immobilization with the forearm across the chest is needed for 2–3 weeks. For the femur, properly applied and supervised Bryant's traction can be used until the fracture is reasonably firm at about 1 week, followed by a further week or two in a plaster spica. Treatment is simple and satisfactory also in a Pavlik harness. If the fracture occurs in a baby who was in the extended breech position in utero, the proximal fragment tends to flex strongly and marked angular malunion will follow if this is not appreciated. Although angular malunions of up to 40° will normally correct quite rapidly with growth, this problem can be avoided by immobilizing the baby in the squat position in a spica cast after 5–7 days of traction.

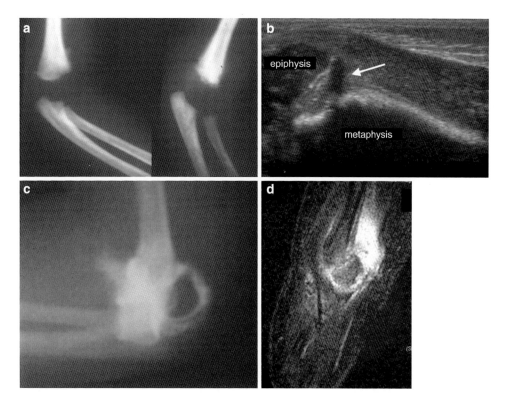

Fig. 5.4 Fracture-separation of distal humeral epiphysis at birth. (**a**) Plain radiograph at 6 days. Early subperiosteal ossification is developing. The alignment is wrong but the lack of epiphyseal ossification makes understanding difficult. (**b**) Ultrasound confirms the displaced epiphysis. (**c**) Lateral view of arthrogram: epiphyseal displacement is even clearer.MRI confirms displacement and demonstrates huge hematoma

Fig. 5.5 Short oblique humeral fracture seen shortly after birth. (**a**) The initial appearance. (**b**) Healing at 3 weeks

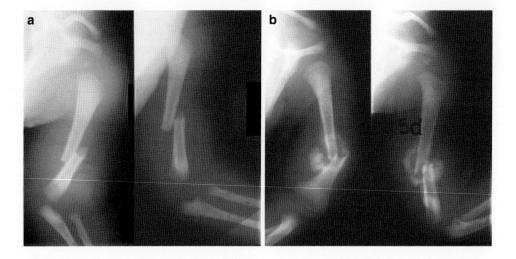

Overlap and angulatory malunion normally correct quite quickly and full functional recovery is the rule. However, rotational malalignment should be corrected whenever possible to prevent long-term abnormality [18].

Proximal Femur

Fracture separation of the upper femoral epiphysis is uncommon but can be confused with developmental dysplasia. The leg lies flexed, abducted, and externally rotated at the hip. There is local swelling and pain on gentle examination. The radiographic appearances suggest congenital dislocation or proximal femoral dysplasia. However, the acetabular appearance is normal (acetabular angle below 30°). The metaphysis tends to buttonhole anteriorly and laterally through the torn periosteum, leaving an intact posterior hinge [19]. Ultrasound will confirm that the femoral head is in the acetabulum and an arthrogram can be carried out if doubt

persists. The displacement can usually be reduced by putting the leg in abduction, internal rotation, and slight flexion. Immobilization in a spica in this position or treatment with overhead traction in abduction minimize the risk of late femoral neck retro-version and coxa vara.

Distal Femur

Separation of the distal chondroepiphysis can occur, particularly after breech delivery (Fig. 5.6). This is usually incomplete and produces a picture similar to that seen in child abuse with varying degrees of periosteal stripping. Assessment of the degree of displacement is easier at the knee than it is at the elbow because the epiphyseal ossific centre is present in most term infants [20]. Differentiation from congenital dislocation (see Chapter 8 of Children's Upper and Lower Limb Orthopaedic Disorders) is usually straightforward (Fig. 42.7).

Fig. 5.6 Fracture separation of distal femoral epiphysis. Ossification makes it easier to appreciate the displacement. (**a**) Lateral and (**b**) AP knee radiographs demonstrate the shear injury

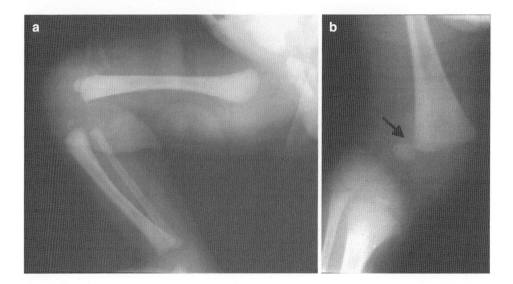

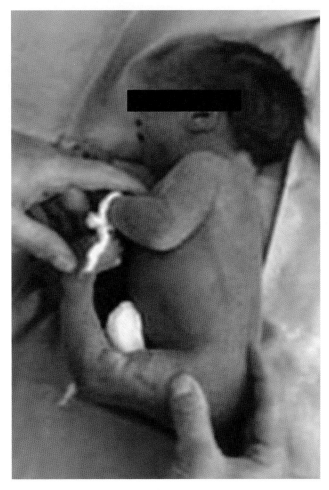

Fig. 5.7 Infant with knee dislocation related to intrauterine position and not to a birth injury

Distal Tibia

Posterior epiphyseal displacement occasionally occurs with hyperflexion of the foot. The deformity is apparent and is associated with swelling and tenderness. It should not be confused with simple equinus deformity. Plain radiographs demonstrate malalignment but the injury is better demonstrated by ultrasound which is also useful to monitor reduction. Healing is accompanied by extensive periosteal new bone. The prognosis is excellent.

Cervical Spine

Cervical cord and cervical vertebral injuries are most likely to occur during breech delivery when there is difficulty with the after-coming head or in vertex deliveries when there is a shoulder dystocia (see Chapter 14).

The historical experiments of Duncan [21] demonstrated that the cervical spine tends to fail when sustained loads of the order of 100 lb (45 kg) are applied. In traction the meninges and the cord usually fail before the vertebrae [22]. Cervical cord injury has been implicated in up to 10% of infant deaths which occur at the time of delivery. Cervical spine injuries are normally associated with marked dystocia and sometimes the obstetrician feels a snap or "give" during traction to deliver the after-coming head in breech deliveries or the shoulder in vertex presentations.

Vertebral injuries do occur [23] and may be associated with respiratory distress or brachial plexus palsy. The mode of vertebral failure is usually a fracture-separation between the body and the physis of the vertebral end plate. Because the facet joints are relatively horizontal in infancy, cervical fractures are both unstable and easily reduced in extension.

The normal failure mode is through the upper vertebral end plate with forward displacement of the more cephalad vertebra at this level. Rarely, the displacement may be posterior with a vertical separation at the body-arch synchondroses.

Because of the relative prominence of the occiput in the infant, babies with cervical spine injuries should be nursed supine on a sponge support with a hollow for the back of the head. If they are nursed on a flat surface, the cervical spine is brought into flexion and displacement at the fracture site increased (see Chapter 14).

Differential Diagnosis of Neonatal Injury

The neonate tends to lie in the fetal flexed posture and, when awake, normal limb mobility is evident. Abnormal immobility of arm or leg is due either to true weakness from brachial plexus or spinal cord injury or to pseudoparalysis which occurs when the limb is painful. In the first few days of life the diagnosis is between plexus injury and clavicular fracture or epiphyseal fracture separation, bearing in mind that both conditions can co-exist. After the first few days, osteomyelitis or septic arthritis must also be considered. Infantile osteomyelitis has a propensity to cause physeal damage with partial growth arrest so that prompt treatment is essential (see Chapter 10 of Children's Upper and Lower Limb Orthopaedic Disorders). Complete cervical spinal cord damage produces tetraplegia and the diagnosis is obvious. Incomplete cord damage may be mistaken for spinal muscular atrophy, myotonia congenita, or hypoxic–ischemic brain damage; it should be appreciated that radiographs are usually normal. Clearly limb weakness may also be caused by cerebral palsy.

Acknowledgment It is a pleasure to record my thanks to Klaus Parsch and David Wilson for some of the images and to Paul Cooper, exemplary photographer, at the Nuffield Orthopaedic Centre NHS Trust.

Part II: Non-Accidental Injuries

Jacqueline Y.Q. Mok

Introduction

Child abuse involves acts of commission or omission which directly or indirectly result in harm to the child and affect its normal development into healthy adulthood. The prevalence is difficult to measure as events tend to be unreported by children and some professionals are reluctant to recognize the nature of the injury. Neglect remains the commonest form of abuse. The phrase "non-accidental injury" (NAI) is used to describe physical abuse in children. Physical abuse includes hitting, shaking, throwing, poisoning, burning or scalding, drowning, and suffocating. It may also result from fabricating or inducing illness in the child.

Most children who have been physically abused present with cutaneous injuries and fractures. If non-accidental injury is not recognized, there is the risk of further injury with significant morbidity and mortality. The risk of subsequent injury may be as high as 20% and of death 5% [24]. Safeguarding children from harm and promoting their well-being is the responsibility of all doctors, whether or not they work directly with children. Therefore all doctors should be familiar with national and local child protection policies and procedures and act on them if there is any suspicion of abuse [25, 26]. Most errors are caused either by not sharing information or by not revising an assessment when new information becomes available.

Doctors working in Accident and Emergency (A & E) departments who see children with fractures regularly miss indicators of abuse. Taitz et al. [27] analyzed the medical records of all children below the age of 3 years who were treated for a long bone fracture in a tertiary children's hospital. The mean age of 100 children who presented with 103 fractures was 21.6 months, with 14 patients younger than 12 months. Thirty-one children were considered to have indicators suspicious of abuse, but only one child was referred to child protection services for further evaluation.

Diagnosis

Recognition

The history of the injury may be inappropriate and may change if the initial explanation is rejected or more injuries come to light. Factors that should alert the clinician to suspect non-accidental injury are the following:

- History which is vague, inconsistent, and discrepant with clinical findings or the child's developmental stage.
- History which is unexplained; the event happened in the absence of witnesses, or a sibling is blamed for the injury.
- Significant delay between injury and seeking medical attention, without credible explanation.
- Evasive or aggressive responses from the parent when details of injury are sought.
- Presence of other injuries.
- Evidence of frank neglect—e.g., non-organic failure to thrive, lack of hygiene.
- Previous concerns regarding child or sibling(s)—e.g., lack of care, unusual injuries, repeated attendances at A&E.

Risk Factors

Child abuse and neglect usually result from interplay between several risk and protective factors. The risk factors identified [28] are shown in Table 5.1. The risk of recurrence following an index incident is high. Hindley et al. [29] reviewed the evidence base for predicting those children at highest risk of recurrent maltreatment. Rates of recurrence were difficult to calculate due to differing follow-up times but ranged from 3.5 to 22.2% at 6 months. The time of greatest risk was the first month after an index episode. Important predictors of recurrence were the number of previous episodes of maltreatment, neglect, parental conflict, and parental mental health problems.

Cutaneous Injuries

Bruises

The commonest non-accidental injury to soft tissues is bruising. Any part of the body is vulnerable. Accidental bruises are related to increased mobility. A systematic review [30] reported accidental bruises in fewer than 1% of babies who were not independently mobile, 17% of infants who were just mobile, 53% of walkers, and the majority of school-aged

Table 5.1 Risk Factors for Child Abuse

Parental background	Socio-economic environment	Family environment	Child characteristics
Young parents	Poverty	High parity	Unintended pregnancy
Low educational attainment	Mother unemployed	Single mother	Low birth weight
Past psychiatric history	Poor social networks	Reported domestic violence	Few positive attributes reported
History of abuse in childhood		Re-ordered family	

Adapted from Sidebotham and Heron [5]

children. Abusive bruises tended to be found away from bony prominences were large, multiple, and occurred in clusters. Commonly affected sites were the head and neck, buttocks, trunk, and arms. Sometimes, a bruise may carry an imprint of the implement used. However, it is not possible to age a bruise accurately, from a description of its color alone, either in vivo or from a photograph [31, 32].

Bites

The characteristic bite mark consists of oval or circular marks which may form two opposing arcs. Teeth marks and ecchymoses may or may not be present. Bites are currently the only abusive injury where the perpetrator may be identified by using DNA technology and dental characteristics. It is therefore essential that clinicians recognize a human bite mark so that referral can be made to a forensic dentist. If there is a delay in obtaining a forensic dental opinion, the bite should be swabbed for saliva and DNA. Photographs should be taken, incorporating a right-angled ruler positioned parallel to the injury. Serial photographs taken at 12–24 h intervals are recommended to assess evolving bite marks [33]. The clinical characteristics which define abusive bites have not been defined [34].

Skeletal Injuries

Studies of the epidemiology of childhood fractures provide useful information on which to base a diagnosis of non-accidental injuries. In a retrospective analysis of 2,198 fractures presenting to one paediatric center in the year 2000, the commonest accidental fractures were found to involve the distal radius and the ulna. [35] The overall mean age of children presenting with fractures was 9.7 years; the incidence increased with age (Table 5.2). Only 27 children (1.2%) sustained more than one fracture. Multiple and unusual fractures should alert the orthopaedic surgeon to the possibility of non-accidental injury.

Non-accidental fractures indicate a serious assault on a child. The prevalence of non-accidental fractures is between 11 and 55% of physically abused children, depending on the age of the population studied. In a comparative study of fracture patterns in accidental and non-accidental injuries, 80% of children with abusive fractures were found to be young (less than 18 months old), whereas 85% of accidental fractures occur in children more than 5 years old. The authors concluded that one in eight children under the age of 18 months who sustains a fracture may be a victim of abuse [36].

In a retrospective analysis of 467 children presenting or referred with a suspicion of non-accidental fractures, 91% were less than 2 years old. [37] The presenting features were often subtle, with medical non-traumatic features (drowsiness, decreased consciousness levels, breathing difficulties, apnea, seizures, vomiting, failure to thrive) and bruises being most common. Eleven children (8%) were brought in dead, mainly from non-accidental head injuries. A total of 1,689 non-accidental fractures were found in 408 children, affecting the long bones (36%), ribs (26%), metaphysis (23%), and skull (15%). About two-thirds of the children had multiple fractures. Isolated long bone fractures involved the femur (25, with 2 metaphyseal fractures), tibia (14, with 5 metaphyseal fractures), humerus (27, with 1 metaphyseal fracture), forearm (9), clavicle (2), and rib (11). Less common fractures involved the scapula, digits, spine, pelvis, and mandible. [37]

Table 5.2 The basic epidemiology of fractures in children by age group

Age group (years)	Prevalence (%)	Incidence/1000/year	Commonest fractures
0–1	2.1	3.6	Clavicle (22.2%) Distal humerus (22.2%)
2–4	11.6	12.9	Distal humerus (22.0%) Distal radius (21.3%)
5–11	51.3	23.2	Distal radius (40.3%) Finger phalanges (14.4%)
12–16	33.8	26.6	Distal radius (28%) Finger phalanges (20.3%)

Adapted from Rennie et al. [12]

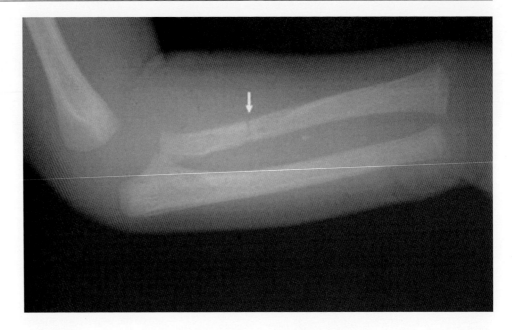

Fig. 5.8 Transverse fracture in the midshaft of radius in a 6-week-old infant admitted with periorbital bruising

Diaphyseal (Long Bone) Fractures

These are the most common inflicted fractures. Typically there is a single rather than multiple fractures and the fracture is diaphyseal rather than metaphyseal [36]. Figs. 5.8, 5.9, and 5.10 show examples of inflicted fractures in infants.

Subperiosteal New Bone Formation (SNBF)

Periosteal elevation with subperiosteal new bone formation may be seen in child abuse [38] as part of the healing process following a fracture or as a non-specific finding in metabolic and infectious conditions. It may be difficult to differentiate from the "physiologic" periosteal reaction

in infants. The "physiological" reaction is usually bilateral, often less than 2 mm in thickness and occurs around the femur. If in doubt, follow-up radiographs help to demonstrate significant changes in traumatic SNBF.

The Classic Metaphyseal Lesion (CML)

Also known as a "bucket handle," "chip," or "corner" fracture, this was regarded as pathognomonic for NAI. It is thought to be produced by shearing, such as when an infant is shaken with the limbs flailing and unsupported [39]. The injuries have been reported to occur accidentally at birth or during physiotherapy to neonates. The CML may be asymptomatic and recent fractures are difficult to visualize

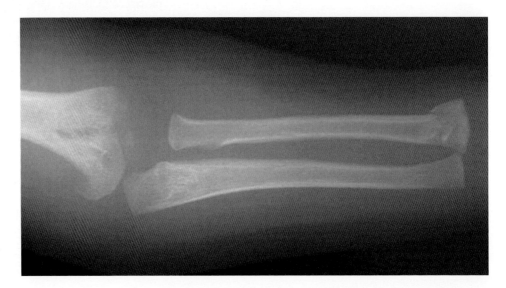

Fig. 5.9 Fractures in right arm—distal radius and ulna, distal humerus—in 20-month-old who presented with facial bruising

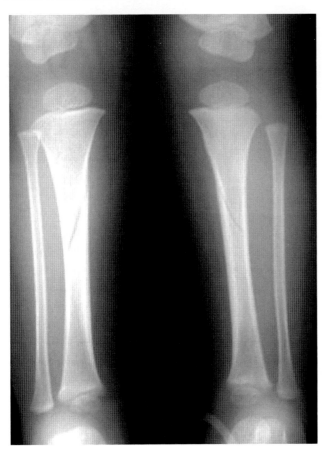

Fig. 5.10 Same infant as in Fig. 5.9, bilateral spiral fractures of tibia found on skeletal survey

radiologically. Appearances depend on the angle at which the radiograph was taken, as well as the stage of healing. Fig. 5.11 illustrates a distal femoral CML in a 6-week-old infant.

Rib Fractures

A systematic review [40] of fractures in child abuse has shown that rib fractures which are found in children without explicit explanation have the highest specificity of abuse. The fractures commonly occur posteriorly at the head–neck junction of the ribs. The detection of occult rib fractures is improved by asking for oblique rib views in the skeletal survey and by another set of views 10–14 days later. Cardio-pulmonary resuscitation (CPR) has often been used in defense argument to explain rib fractures in the young child found collapsed. Maguire and colleagues [41] reviewed 427 studies to establish the evidence base for this opinion. Only six studies met their strict methodological criteria and included 923 children who had had CPR performed by both medical and non-medical personnel. Rib fractures were found to be rare (<2%) after CPR. When they did occur, they were often multiple and found to be anterior.

Skull Fractures

Between 5 and 10% of children who have been abused have skull fractures, which tend to be complex (depressed,

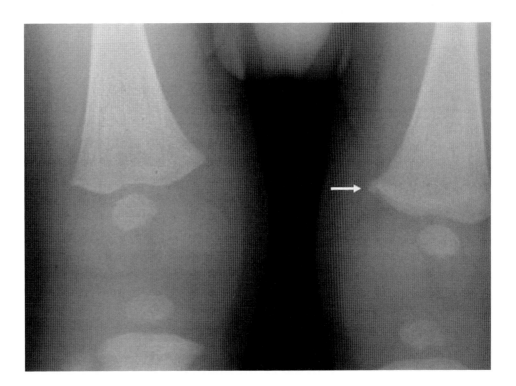

Fig. 5.11 Metaphyseal fracture at the distal end of the femur

compound, or comminuted) and involve more than a single cranial bone. Diastasis of fracture margins is sometimes seen ("growing" fracture), usually in association with an underlying dural injury [42]. Skull fractures are the result of a direct blow or part of shaking which ends with impact. Further neuroimaging [computed tomography (CT) or magnetic resonance imaging (MRI) brain scan] should always be considered in young infants who present with skull fractures.

Assessment

A fracture, like any other injury, should never be interpreted in isolation. It must always be assessed in the context of the medical and social history, developmental stage, and any explanation given. Child abuse should be suspected under the following circumstances:

- Child less than 18 months old.
- Fracture inconsistent with child's developmental stage.
- Multiple fractures of different ages in the absence of an adequate explanation.
- Rib fractures in children with normal bones and no history of major trauma.
- Fractured femur in a pre-mobile child.

The investigation and management of a possibly harmed child must be in the same systematic and rigorous manner as would be appropriate for the investigation and management of any other potentially fatal disease [43]. The doctor must be aware of the referral pathways to senior colleagues with the specialist skills necessary to help assess whether the child has been abused. However, it is not necessary to make a firm diagnosis of child abuse before referral to the statutory agencies (social services or police).

Record keeping is vital and must be contemporaneous, comprehensive, and legible. Negative as well as positive findings must be recorded. Any statements from the child or the parent must be written down verbatim. Body charts are helpful for documenting injuries. Photographs are useful.

Inter-Agency Cooperation

The mechanisms for investigating potential child abuse vary considerably around the world. A structured and validated approach is essential both to protect the child and to avoid inappropriate censure of the parents. When non-accidental injury is suspected, it is necessary to consider both the injuries themselves and co-existing forms of abuse. In the United Kingdom, the Child Protection Register should be checked by telephoning social services. Local as well as

national procedures and guidelines must be followed to ensure the child's safety [25, 26].

A multi-agency child protection enquiry should be commenced by contacting the social services department who should in turn discuss the case with the police. Referrals should be followed up in writing within 24 h. Social services have a statutory responsibility to make enquiries when concerns are expressed about a child, while police have a duty to investigate. In the United Kingdom, a multi-agency meeting (child protection conference), attended by the parents and all concerned, is the forum where professionals decide, based on the available information, whether the child has suffered harm. If so, the child is placed on the Child Protection Register and a Child Protection Plan agreed with the parents to ensure the safety and well-being of their child. Risks to other children living in the same household must also be considered during the case conference.

Differential Diagnosis

It is important to exclude other causes which might have contributed to the injury. An underlying medical condition might be responsible for fractures, such as the following:

- Normal variant/physiological finding, e.g., subperiosteal new bone formation.
- Accidental injury.
- Birth injury in a young infant. Most fractures sustained at birth heal within a few weeks. Obstetric and neonatal records should be checked.
- Bone disease, e.g., osteogenesis imperfecta, osteopenia of prematurity, rickets, copper deficiency, osteomyelitis, scurvy, and metastatic lesions.

However, it is important to remember that abuse may co-exist with an underlying medical problem.

Investigations

High-quality radiographs and interpretation by a skilled paediatric radiologist will increase fracture detection rate. The British Society of Paediatric Radiology has established standards for skeletal imaging in cases of suspected non-accidental injury [44]. In children under 2 years of age where physical abuse is suspected, skeletal surveys should be mandatory. Predictive factors which might guide clinical practice include the age of the child (younger than 12 months) and the type of presenting injury (overt fracture or head injury) [45]. However, no single radiological investigation (skeletal survey or bone scan) has been found to identify all fractures. Bone scans will identify acute fractures not seen easily on skeletal surveys but may miss skull fractures. Diagnostic accuracy is increased if all skeletal surveys include oblique views of the ribs, with follow-up films to evaluate suspicious findings [46]. Criminal investigators often rely on the radiological dating of injuries to exclude or identify perpetrators. Didactic statements are often forthcoming on the date of a bone injury: the primary evidence for these statements is lacking. Although a recent fracture can be distinguished from an old one, the dating of the age of a fracture based on its pattern of healing is imprecise [47].

The two most common causes of bone fragility in infancy are osteopenia of prematurity and osteogenesis imperfecta. In pre-term infants, fractures associated with osteopenia tend to occur in the first two years of life. Risk factors which predispose to fractures are cholestatic jaundice, intravenous nutrition for more than 3 weeks, chronic lung disease, diuretic treatment for longer than 2 weeks, and physiotherapy [48]. The controversial entity of "temporary brittle bone disease" has been dismissed by the European Society of Paediatric Radiology as a possible explanation for fractures in children [49].

Apart from careful history taking and examination, blood must be taken to evaluate biochemical markers of bone disease (calcium, phosphate, alkaline phosphatase, copper, magnesium, fasting 25-hydroxyvitamin D, and parathyroid hormone levels). It is helpful to discuss with an experienced paediatric radiologist the need for further radiological investigations, e.g., special views and MRI scans. Where a non-accidental fracture is suspected in a child under 2 years of age, a full skeletal survey must be performed to exclude occult fractures. Repeat radiographs of doubtful areas should be obtained 1–2 weeks later to identify callus (which helps with approximate dating of injury) and to demonstrate previously occult injuries. While a laboratory diagnosis of osteogenesis imperfecta can be made from a skin biopsy (biochemical analysis of collagen species and mutation analysis of RNA) or from a blood sample (mutation analysis of DNA), both take a long time and are not readily available: adequate samples of skin in infants are technically difficult to obtain and the investigations are available only in specialist centers. No clear guidelines are available regarding the utility of these investigations in suspected non-accidental injury. Furthermore, the positive predictive value of these tests has not been defined.

Conclusion

Awareness that abuse may underlie injury is essential. Although more common in the financially deprived, it occurs throughout society and in communities world over. Nearly 50% occur in infants under 1 year. Toddlers, children, and adolescents are equally affected and in the last group neurological or psychiatric problems are common [50]. In the United States, child maltreatment is estimated to occur in 15–42 cases per 1,000 children and over one million children each year are the substantiated victims [51]. In the United Kingdom, a national study of young people estimated that 1 in 4 children experienced one or more forms of physical violence during childhood. Of this 25% of children, the majority had experienced some degree of physical abuse by parents or carers [52]. Although the history and findings may be suggestive of abuse, no fracture pattern is pathognomonic.

References

1. Xian CJ, Foster BK. The biologic aspects of children's fractures. In: Rockwood CA, Wilkins KE, Beaty JH, Kasser JR, eds. Rockwood and Wilkins' Fractures in Children, 6th ed. Philadelphia: Lippincott, Williams and Wilkins; 2006:21–50.
2. Shapiro F, Holtrop ME, Glimcher MJ. Organisation and cellular biology of the perichondrial ossification groove of Ranvier. A morphological study in rabbits. J Bone Joint Surg 1977; 59A: 703–23.
3. Marks SC Jr. The structure and developmental contexts of skeletal injury. In: Kleinman PK, ed. Diagnostic Imaging of Child Abuse, 2nd ed. St. Louis: Mosby; 1988:2–7.
4. Curry JD, Butler G. The mechanical properties of bone tissue in children. J Bone Joint Surg 1975; 57A: 810–14.
5. Thorndike A, Pierce FR. Fractures in the newborn. A plea for adequate treatment. New England J Med 1936; 215:1013–18.
6. Rubin A. Birth injuries: incidence, mechanisms and end results. Obstet Gynecol 1964; 23:218–21.
7. Wickstrom I, Axelsson D, Bergstrom R, Meirik O. Traumatic injury in large-for-dates infants. Acta Obstet Gynecol Scand 1988; 67:259–64.
8. Gresham EL. Birth Trauma. Ped Clin North Am 1977; 22:317–28.
9. Nadas S, Gudinchet F, Capasso P, Reinberg O. Predisposing factors in obstetric fractures. Skeletal Radiol 1993; 22:195–8.
10. Oppenheim WL, Davis A, Growden WA, et al. Clavicle fracture in the newborn. Clin Orthop 1990; 250:176–80.
11. Greenwald AG, Schute PC, Shively JL. Brachial plexus palsy. A 10 year report on the incidence and prognosis. J Ped Orthop 1984; 4:689–92.
12. Owen R. Congenital pseudarthrosis of the clavicle. J Bone Joint Surg 1970; 52B: 644–52.
13. Lemperg R, Liliequist B. Dislocation of the proximal epiphysis of the humerus in newborns: report of two cases and discussion of diagnostic criteria. Acta Ped Scand 1970; 59:373–80.
14. Broker FH, Burbach T. Ultrasonic diagnosis of separation of the proximal humeral epiphysis in the newborn. J Bone Joint Surg 1990; 72A: 187–91.
15. Bayne O, Rang M. Medial dislocation of the radial head following breech delivery: a case report and review of the literature. J Ped Orthop 1984; 4:485–7.
16. Downs DM, Wirth CR. Fracture of the distal humeral chondroepiphysis in the neonate. Clin Orthop 1982; 169:155–58.
17. Barrett WP, Almquist EA, Staheli LT. Fracture separation of the distal humeral epiphysis in the newborn. J Ped Orthop 1984; 4:617–19.

18. Hagglund G, Hansson LI, Wiberg G. Correction of deformity after femoral birth fracture. 16 year follow-up. Acta Orthop Scand 1988; 59:333–35.

19. Ogden JA, Lee KE, Rudicel SA, Pelker RR. Proximal femoral epiphysis in the neonate. J Ped Orthop 1984; 4:282–92.

20. Hensinger RN. Standards in Pediatric Orthopaedics. New York: Raven Press; 1986:284.

21. Byers RK. Spinal-cord injuries during birth. Dev Med Child Neurol 1975; 17:103–10.

22. Lanska MJ, Roessman U, Wiznitzer M. Magnetic resonance imaging in cervical cord birth injury. Pediatrics 1990; 85:760–5.

23. Stanley P, Duncan AW, Isaacson J, Isaacson JS. Radiology of fracture-dislocation of the cervical spine during delivery. Am J Radiol 1985; 145:621–5.

24. Morse CW, Sahler OJZ, Friedman SB. A three-year follow up study of abused and neglected children. Am J Dis Child 1970; 120:439–46.

25. Department of Health. Working together to safeguard children. London: The Stationery Office, 2006. At: http://www.everychild matters.gov.uk/_files/AE53C8F9D7AEB1B23E403514A6C1B17D. pdf. Accessed 15 October 2008.

26. Protecting Children and Young People. Framework for Standards. The Scottish Executive, Edinburgh 2004. At: http://www.scotland. gov.uk/Resource/Doc/1181/0008818.pdf. Accessed 15 October 2008.

27. Taitz J, Moran K, O'Meara M. Long bone fractures in children under 3 years of age: Is abuse being missed in Emergency Department presentations? J Pediatr Child Health 2004; 40:170–4.

28. Sidebotham P, Heron J. Child maltreatment in the "children of the nineties": A cohort study of risk factors. Child Abuse Negl 2006; 30:497–522.

29. Hindley N, Ramchandani PG, Jones DPH. Risk factors for recurrence of maltreatment: a systematic review. Arch Dis Child 2006; 91:744–52.

30. Maguire S, Mann MK, Sibert J, Kemp A. Are there patterns of bruising in childhood which are diagnostic or suggestive of abuse? A systematic review. Arch Dis Child 2005; 90:182–6.

31. Maguire S, Mann MK, Sibert J, Kemp A. Can you age bruises accurately in children? A systematic review. Arch Dis Child 2005; 90:187–9.

32. Munang LA, Leonard PA, Mok J. Lack of agreement on colour description between clinicians examining childhood bruising. J Clin Foren Med 2002; 9:171–4.

33. British Association of Forensic Odontology. Guidelines Bitemark Methodology. 2001. At: http://www.forensicdentistryonline. org/forensic_pages_1/bitemarkguide.htm. Accessed 15 October 2008.

34. Kemp A, Maguire SA, Sibert J, et al. Can we identify abusive bites in children? Arch Dis Child 2006; 91:951.

35. Rennie L, Court-Brown CM, Mok JYQ, Beattie TF. The epidemiology of fractures in children. Injury 2007; 38:913–22.

36. Worlock P, Stower M, Barbor P. Patterns of fractures in accidental and non-accidental injury in children: a comparative study. Br Med J 1986; 293:100–2.

37. Carty H, Pierce A. Non-accidental injury: a retrospective analysis of a large cohort. Europ Radiol 2002; 12:2919–25.

38. Kleinman PK. Skeletal trauma: general considerations. In: Kleinman PK, ed. Diagnostic Imaging of Child Abuse, 2nd edition. St. Louis: Mosby; 1998:8–25.

39. Kleinman PK, Marks SC, Blackbourne B. The metaphyseal lesion in abused infants: a radiologic–histologic study. Am J Roentgenol 1986; 146:895–905.

40. Kemp AM, Dunstan F, Harrison S, et al. Patterns of skeletal fractures in child abuse: systemic review. BMJ 2008; 337:a1518.

41. Maguire S, Mann M, John N, et al. Does cardiopulmonary resuscitation cause rib fractures in children? A systematic review. Child Abuse Negl 2006; 30:739–51.

42. Hobbs CJ. Skull fracture and the diagnosis of abuse. Arch Dis Child 1984; 59:246–52.

43. Report of an Inquiry into the death of Victoria Climbie. Lord Laming. London: The Stationery Office; 2003.

44. British Society of Paediatric Radiology. NAI standard for skeletal surveys. At: http://www.bspr.org.uk/nai.htm. Accessed 10 November 2008.

45. Day F, Clegg S, McPhillips M, Mok J. A retrospective case series of skeletal surveys in children with suspected non-accidental injury. J Clin For Med 2006; 13:55–9.

46. Kemp AM, Butler A, Morris S, et al. Which radiological investigations should be performed to identify fractures in suspected child abuse? Clin Radiol 2006; 61:723–36.

47. Prosser I, Maguire S, Harrison S, et al. How old is this fracture? Radiological dating of fractures in children: a systematic review. Am J Roentgenol 2005; 184:1282–6.

48. Bishop N, Sprigg A, Dalton A. Unexplained fractures in infancy: looking for fragile bones. Arch Dis Child 2007; 92:251–6.

49. Mendelson KL. Critical review of "temporary brittle bone disease." Pediatr Radiol 2005; 35:1036–40.

50. Loder RT, Feinberg JR. Orthopedic injuries in children with nonaccidental trauma. J Pediatr Orthop 2007; 27:421–6

51. Kocher MS, Kasser JR. Orthopaedic aspects of child abuse. J Am Acad Orthop Surg. 2000; 8:10–20.

52. Cawson P, Wattam C, Brooker S, Kelly G. Child maltreatment in the United Kingdom: a study of the prevalence of child abuse and neglect, 2000. London: NSPCC. ISBN: 1842280066.

Chapter 6

Fractures Around the Shoulder and the Humerus

J.B. Hunter

Clavicle Fractures

Etiology

Fractures of the clavicle are seen extremely commonly in the children's fracture clinic. The vast majority are of the diaphysis and are caused by a fall on the outstretched hand. These low-energy fractures occur in children who have an excellent potential for remodeling. After 7–10 days a mass forms over the affected clavicle: this represents a healing fracture callus and disappears within another 2–3 weeks when the fracture has stabilized.

Treatment

Conservative management with a sling or a figure-of-eight bandage is the traditional treatment. The figure-of-eight bandage has some theoretical advantages in that it braces the shoulders back and preserves clavicular length. In practice the bandage and even the commercial varieties loosen easily and children find them rather uncomfortable. There is no evidence that the figure-of-eight bandage offers any superior analgesia and therefore our practice has been to use a simple sling worn underneath the clothes [1]. The sling or figure-of-eight bandage needs to be worn for 10–20 days depending on the age of the child and the configuration of the fracture. No further radiographs are required and we do not routinely follow these patients up. We allow them to remove their own sling or figure-of-eight bandage and return to normal activities 3 weeks after injury (Fig. 6.1).

J.B. Hunter (✉)
Departments of Trauma and Orthopaedics, Nottingham University Hospital, Nottingham, UK

Very occasionally diaphyseal fractures of the clavicle require internal fixation because of patient factors such as polytrauma, floating shoulder, or neurovascular injury. In these situations stabilization is advantageous, and may be done either by plating or more commonly with elastic stable intramedullary nailing [2].

Obstetrical Clavicle Fracture

In obstetric and neonatal practice fractures of the clavicle are associated with shoulder dystocia and brachial plexus palsy. The fracture itself rarely requires any active intervention but the child requires follow-up in order to establish that any tendency to underuse in the arm is related to the fracture rather than any underlying palsy [3].

Fracture Dislocations of the Medial and Lateral Ends of the Clavicle

Fractures and dislocations of the medial and distal ends of the clavicle are unusual. There are physes at each end of the clavicle. Increased mobility after trauma that appears to be caused by a dislocation is in fact a growth plate injury in which the metaphysis can rupture out of the periosteal sleeve. These need to be recognized because, although the fractures will heal protected by a figure-of-eight splint, there will be massive sub-periosteal new bone formation, which may or may not fully remodel. At the distal end of the clavicle the periosteal sleeve remains attached both to the capsule of the acromioclavicular joint and the coraco-clavicular ligaments. In adolescents stabilization may be achieved by careful periosteal repair. K-wire fixation is never advised to avoid possible migration [4]. At the medial end of the clavicle reduction, periosteal suture is necessary if a fracture has displaced posteriorly and compressed underlying structures causing stridor and/or dysphagia [5].

Fig. 6.1 Clavicle healing and remodeling. Courtesy of K. Parsch

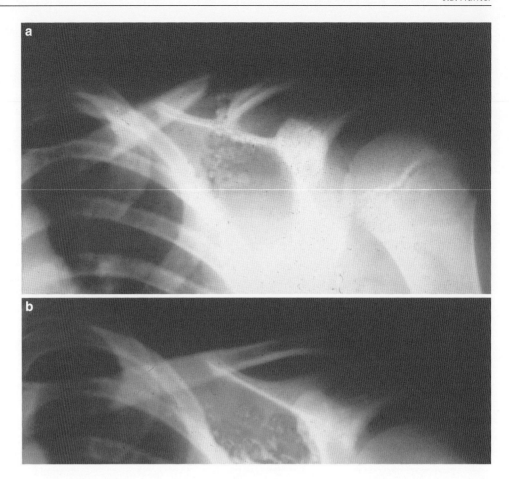

Fractures of the Scapula

Fractures of the scapula are unusual in paediatric practice and body fractures are virtually only seen in the multi-injured. There are multiple secondary ossification centers in the scapula, which can be mistaken for fractures, but are also potential sites of weakness, particularly in teenagers. Fractures at the junction of the body of the scapula and the coracoid process do occur and are frequently missed. Similarly, the apophyses around the acromion are occasionally diagnosed as fractures in cases of bruised shoulder.

Fractures of the Proximal Humerus

Fractures of the proximal humerus are fairly uncommon with an incidence of 1–2 per 1000 (about 5% of paediatric fractures) [6].

Classification

Fractures of the proximal humerus are best classified using the AO paediatric fracture classification [7], all classifiable within the sections 11 E. or 11 M. The different fracture types

are shown in Fig. 6.2. The epiphyseal fracture types follow the Salter–Harris classification (e.g., 11 E/2) but also have a category for flake fractures (11 E/8). For metaphyseal fractures only type 11 M/2 (torus, buckle, or greenstick fractures) and type 11 M/3 (complete fractures) are seen (Fig. 6.2).

Birth Fractures of the Proximal Humerus

Physeal fractures of the proximal humerus occur in obstetric practice and, because the ossification center of the humeral head has not appeared, tend to be misdiagnosed as congenital dislocations of the humerus. The diagnosis can be established either by arthrogram or more conveniently by ultrasound, which does not require an anesthetic [8]. Once it is established that the head is in the socket no treatment is required beyond a body bandage for analgesia (see Chapter 5).

Proximal Humerus Fracture of the Older Child

In older children direct or indirect trauma may cause the fracture. Because of the thick periosteum and the proximity to the physis there is an enormous potential for healing.

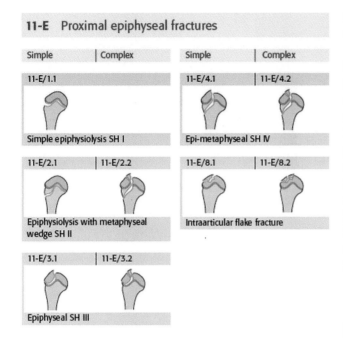

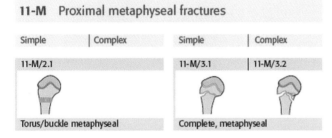

Fig. 6.2 Classification of proximal humeral fractures. From: Slongo T, Audigé L, AO Classification Group. AO Pediatric Comprehensive Classification of Long Bone Fractures (PCCF) Brochure. Davos, Switzerland: AO Publishing; 2007

Remodeling of the proximal humerus occurs more readily than in any other bone. Fractures of the proximal humerus have been described as the most overtreated fracture in the body: Mercer Rang stated that bayonet apposition of the fracture fragments could be accepted at all times, provided 2 years of growth remained [9].

In older children physeal fractures are most commonly Salter–Harris 1 or 2 fractures; intra-articular growth plate injuries are extremely rare. These latter need to be accurately reduced and fixed to allow early mobilization, but the more common extra-articular injuries rarely require operative treatment; there is some evidence that, far from improving the results, operation is associated with an increased rate of complications in the management of these fractures [10]. Although interposition of the biceps tendon has been described in children's fractures, this is rare [11]. More commonly the fracture heals and remodels perfectly, despite significant displacement. Displaced metaphyseal fractures of

the proximal humerus remodel as well as physeal fractures and a conservative approach is appropriate.

If fracture fixation is required because of associated injuries, then elastic nailing is much more elegant than percutaneous K-wire fixation, which risks migration and prevents early mobilization. However, just because this is an elegant technique does not mean that it should be used frequently. If elastic nailing is the chosen management, then technique preferred is retrograde. The starting point is on the lateral supracondylar ridge where two separate holes are made for the nails. The first nail is inserted in a C-shape, the second nail in an S-shape to allow the nail points to diverge in the humeral head. Reduction by the nails is controlled on the image intensifier. Pendulum movements are allowed immediately, with full active mobilization at 7–10 days [12, 13] (Fig. 6.3).

Fractures of the Humerus Shaft

Classification

Plastic deformation and greenstick fractures of the humeral shaft are rare. The main codes for these fractures are therefore 12 D/4 (transverse fractures) and 12 D/5 (oblique or spiral fractures). Fractures of the humeral shaft are rare in children but more common in adolescents with higher energy injuries.

In children the most important aspect of humeral shaft fractures to recognize is the non-accidental injury. A humeral shaft fracture in a child younger than 2 years has been identified as the fracture that is likely to be inflicted, particularly if the fracture pattern is spiral. This information came from a large study of children's fractures in Nottingham, and has been challenged since, but certainly a fracture of the humerus shaft in a non-walking child is highly abnormal and worthy of investigation [14–16].

Treatment

These fractures can generally be managed non-operatively as both healing and remodeling are excellent in children. Initial management should be with a collar and cuff or a hanging cast to allow the weight of the elbow to straighten the humerus. This can be augmented by a sugar tong splint or a coaptation splint. If the physes are open, remodeling is excellent and non-union unlikely. Conservative management of the humeral shaft requires immobilization and splintage for 3–6 weeks depending on the age of the child. Physiotherapy

Fig. 6.3 (**a** and **b**) Fully displaced fracture of the proximal humerus in a 14-year-old girl nearing skeletal maturity. (**c**) and (**d**) Similar fracture in another teenaged girl, stabilized by ESIN. Courtesy of K. Parsch

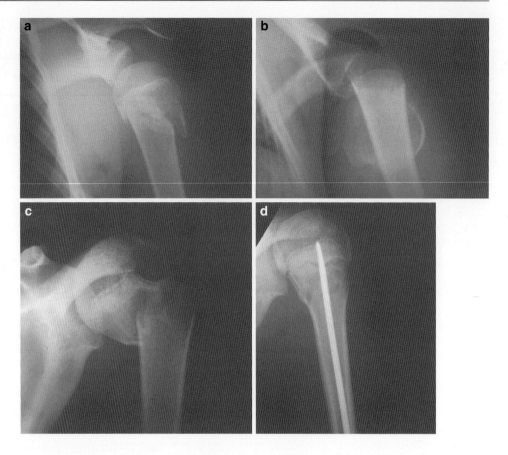

is rarely required, as stiffness of either shoulder or elbow is uncommon.

Injury to the radial nerve in conjunction with the humeral shaft fracture is less common in children than in adults; the norm is for spontaneous resolution and surgical exploration is generally not indicated. Exceptions might be fracture patterns highly suggestive of a laceration to the radial nerve and the onset of a nerve lesion following manipulation or closed surgery.

Indications for surgical stabilization of the humeral shaft are only relative: neurovascular injury, open fractures, and multiple injuries. Pathological fractures secondary to simple bone cysts are well treated by elastic nailing as it allows an earlier return to activities and promotes cyst healing. Fractures of the lower diaphysis or the junction of the shaft and metaphysis are also a relative indication of surgical treatment as residual angulation at this level can lead to functional problems. The most common surgical treatment is by elastic nailing. If the fracture is of the midshaft then elastic nailing should be done from the distal end of the humerus using the technique described above. If the fracture is off the distal third of the humerus, then the nailing should be antegrade from a start point in the region of the deltoid tuberosity [12, 13] (Figs. 6.4 and 6.5).

Fractures of the Distal Humerus

Supracondylar Fractures

The peak ages when supracondylar fractures occur is between 5–7 years. Traditionally, boys have a higher incidence for this fracture than girls, outnumbering girls by about 3:2 [17]. Almost all supracondylar fractures are caused by accidental trauma. A fall from a height such as a bed or furniture in small children or monkey bars or swings in kindergarten and school-age children is a common cause for the injury.

Classification

In the first instance supracondylar fractures should be classified as either extension or flexion types, depending on the angulation or displacement of the distal fragment. Only 5% of displaced supracondylar fractures are of the flexion type; they are difficult to manage and will be considered separately.

The supracondylar fracture is a metaphyseal fracture and the primary code in the AO classification is 13 M/3 (complete

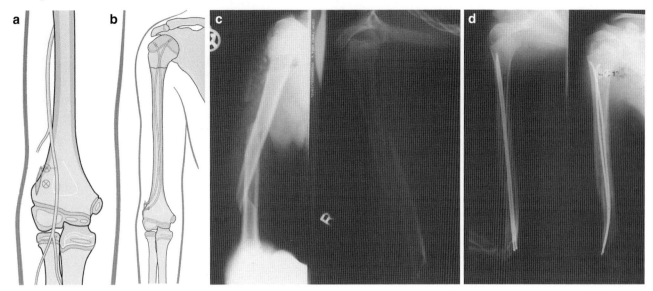

Fig. 6.4 (**a**) Start points for elastic nailing of the humeral shaft or neck. (**b**) Configuration of elastic nails in humeral nailing. From: Dietz H-G, Schmittenbecher P, Slongo T. AO Manual of Fracture Management: Elastic Stable Intramedullary nailing (ESIN) in Children. Davos, Switzerland: AO Publishing; 2006. (**c**) Spiral fracture of the humerus in a 12-year-old boy. Courtesy of K.Parsch. (**d**) Same fracture stabilized by ESIN and healing

Fig. 6.5 Pathological fracture through a simple bone cyst leading to cyst healing at 18 months

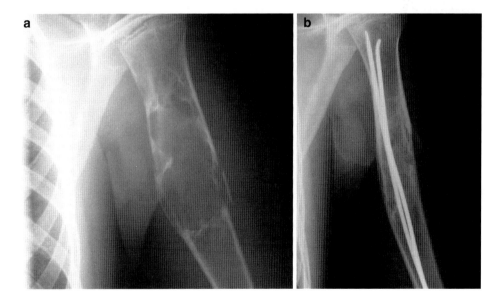

metaphyseal fracture of the distal humerus). The standard English language classification of extension supracondylar fractures is that of Gartland [18], most simply described in three types:

I. Undisplaced fractures.
II. Fractures that are angulated/displaced into extension with an intact posterior cortex.
III. Displaced fractures (Fig. 6.6)

This classification has been validated and shown to perform reasonably well in terms of inter- and intra-observer error. Over time, various authors have added to this classification. Mubarak and Davids described a variant of the undisplaced fracture with comminution or collapse of the medial column [19]. This fracture is certainly unstable with the potential to collapse into varus but is nearly always angulated at initial presentation and therefore not truly undisplaced.

Wilkins described two types of the displaced fracture, the postero-medial and postero-lateral, noting that the latter was much more likely to cause injury to the brachial artery and median nerve [20]. The distinction is more useful if the displacement is incomplete rather than complete, when the distal fragment is fully mobile in all directions.

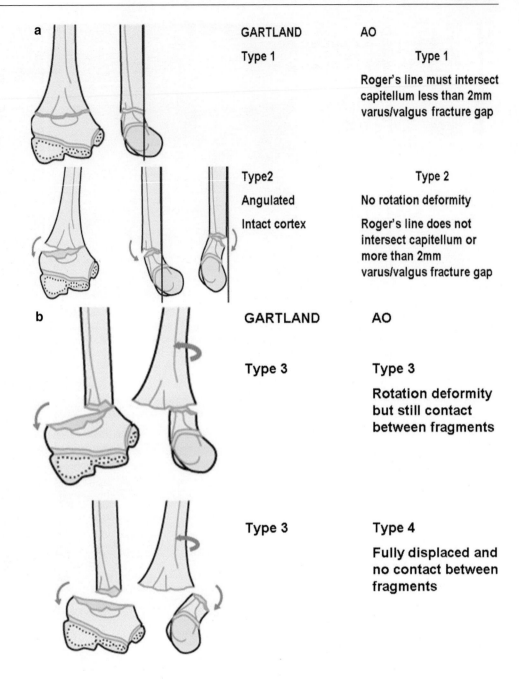

Fig. 6.6 AO and Gartland classification methods for supracondylar fractures. From: Slongo T, Audigé L, AO Classification Group. AO Pediatric Comprehensive Classification of Long Bone Fractures (PCCF) Brochure. Davos, Switzerland: AO Publishing; 2007

GARTLAND	AO
Type 1	Type 1
	Roger's line must intersect capitellum less than 2mm varus/valgus fracture gap
Type2	Type 2
Angulated	No rotation deformity
Intact cortex	Roger's line does not intersect capitellum or more than 2mm varus/valgus fracture gap
GARTLAND	AO
Type 3	Type 3
	Rotation deformity but still contact between fragments
Type 3	Type 4
	Fully displaced and no contact between fragments

In Central Europe, von Laer introduced the concept of rotational failure [21]. In his classification, type 1 was undisplaced, type 2 angulated but with no rotation of the distal fragment, type 3 displaced by rotation of the distal fragment but still in contact between the main fragments, and type 4 fully displaced with no contact between the fragments. Initial attempts to validate this by the AO classification group showed poor reliability, interestingly because of the lack of definition of *undisplaced* [7]. Each modification, therefore, may make Gartland's classification less reproducible.

Treatment

The purpose of classification is mainly to guide treatment which allows Gartland's original classification to remain very useful.

Type I undisplaced supracondylar fractures can be treated in a sling or collar and cuff and need only 3 weeks treatment.

Type II fractures with posterior angulation (apex anterior) should be manipulated under general anesthesia and placed in full flexion. If the reduction is successful the fracture should be stabilized by crossed K-wires. Once stabilized, the position of full flexion can be avoided. Full flexion supposedly predisposes to elevated compartment pressures in the forearm [22], although compartment pressure studies performed by Clavert et al. suggest this may not be the case [23].

Type III fully displaced fractures should not be treated by manipulation and immobilization alone as the success rate is only just over 60%. Chinese authors have described treating the displaced fracture in an extension plaster, taking care to correct varus and valgus, but ignoring any posterior displacement [24]. Traction is still used successfully in some British hospitals [25, 26]. This is time-consuming, but avoids some of the complications associated with percutaneous pinning.

Reduction of the displaced supracondylar fracture is achieved by traction and disimpaction followed by the correction of any medial or lateral displacement. The distal fragment is "thumbed" into place as the elbow is flexed.

One of the controversies in managing these fractures is the configuration of the wires that should be used. Higher rates of ulnar nerve injury have been reported using the typical crossed wire configuration [27]. Multiple wires inserted from the lateral side avoid this complication but are less stable [28]. Excellent results have been reported using two or three lateral wires and obeying these rules [29] (Figs. 6.7 and 6.8):

(1) The wires should be at least 2 mm in diameter.
(2) The wires should diverge to engage both medial and lateral columns.
(3) The medial wire should engage all four cortices at the olecranon fossa.
(4) The construct should be tested for stability in rotation on the table [30].

Many surgeons continue to use crossed wires for stability [31]. Recently, ascending and descending wires inserted from a lateral approach have been shown to provide excellent stability [32]. Ulnar nerve injury can be avoided by inserting the medial wire with the elbow extended as recommended by Rang, and by examining the contralateral elbow for subluxation of the ulnar nerve in flexion and extension.

Alternative methods to stabilize supracondylar fractures include down-going elastic nailing and external fixation. Anterograde elastic nailing was described in Nancy [13]. It has the advantage that the implant is entirely internal and does not cross the joint. This minimizes the need for external protection and allows early mobilization [33]. The disadvantages are that the technique is technically demanding and almost impossible to achieve without two image intensifiers at 90° to each other. In very few units is this standard treatment but it is useful for fractures that are slightly more proximal at the diaphyseal/metaphyseal border. External fixation is a well-described method of stabilizing osteotomies

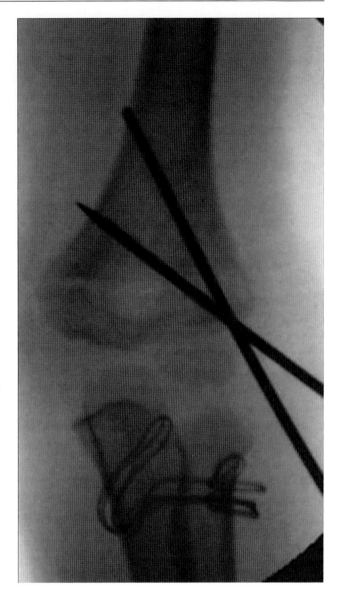

Fig. 6.7 Supracondylar fracture pinned with lateral wires. Courtesy Richard Reynolds

of the distal humerus and may be useful for very unstable or open fractures [34].

Neurovascular Injury

Supracondylar humeral fractures in children generate anxiety and excitement, particularly among trainees and adult surgeons who are exposed to the fracture infrequently. The feared complications are vascular and neural injury. Injury to the brachial artery can be direct laceration, interruption through kinking, vascular spasm, or intimal tear. The consequence of any of these injuries is a compartment syndrome of the flexor compartment of the forearm, which, if untreated,

Fig. 6.8 Typical AO type 4
(Gartland 3) displaced
supracondylar fracture, reduced
and stabilized with crossed
K-wires

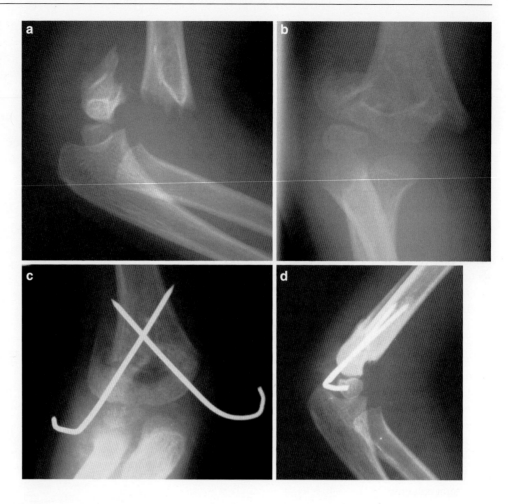

leads to ischemic contracture and severe loss of function in the wrist and hand. Re-establishing the flow in the brachial artery is not the most important aspect of treatment as there is an excellent collateral circulation and symptoms of claudication of the forearm muscles are extremely rare in follow-up studies. The important thing is to monitor, diagnose, and if necessary treat the incipient compartment syndrome by fasciotomy [35].

Management of the Vascular Injury

Assessing vascular status following supracondylar fracture requires examination of three things: the pulse, the capillary return, and the amount of pain from and activity in the forearm muscles. The pulse and the capillary return give information on the state of circulation to the extremity.

If the hand is *white and pulseless* then circulation must be restored [36]. This situation arises most frequently either when the fracture is severely displaced prior to manipulation, or immediately after a reduction maneuver, indicating that the artery has been trapped in or close to the fracture

site. In the first circumstance the action should be gentle provisional reduction, straightening the arm without attempting to definitively reduce the fracture. This should be done in the emergency department under appropriate analgesia. In the second situation, the immediate action should be to re-displace the fracture to see if circulation is restored. Exploration of the artery is likely to be required to prevent it from being entrapped in the fracture when it is reduced for a second time. The white, pulseless hand is, however, fortunately quite rare.

The *pink pulseless* hand is, by contrast, much more common: in our series of supracondylar fractures treated on traction, the pink pulseless hand occurred in more than 10% of cases [37]. If the hand is pink with satisfactory capillary return then the circulation to the extremity is adequate. The necessity is then to prevent a compartment syndrome and ischemic contracture. The normal values of forearm compartment pressure in the young child are not well established. Therefore, the compartment syndrome can only be diagnosed clinically, waking the child up and assessing movements and stretch pain. The vast majority of patients (100% in our series) with a pink pulseless hand recover completely, without exploration of the artery [36]. Protocols that demand exploration of the artery are over-invasive [38]. Exploration is, however, warranted in some situations:

(1) There is a block to accurate reduction.
(2) There is a loss of pulse, accompanied by a nerve injury, particularly of the median or anterior interosseous nerves.
(3) There is severe, disproportionate pain with an accurately reduced and stabilized fracture.

Exploration of the artery may yield a variety of findings. In the most extreme situation, the artery is divided or lacerated, and there is severe local bleeding, which is a potent cause of the compartment syndrome. In this situation, the artery should be repaired using a vein graft [39]. This should be accompanied by forearm fasciotomies. An intimal tear may cause re-occlusion of the artery and the recommendation is that a vein patch be applied.

The more common situation is that the artery is found intact, but collapsed. The collapse may be secondary to vascular spasm caused by direct pressure or to an intimal tear. If the artery is collapsed over an extensive segment the child's blood pressure may not be sufficient to reinflate it. Direct re-inflation is recommended, using a syringe of saline [40].

Flexion Supracondylar Fractures

In this much rarer fracture type, the distal fragment is displaced anteriorly. Generally, the fracture is much more unstable, and conservative methods are difficult to pursue essentially because the elbow must be held fully straight to keep the fracture reduced. This makes closed reduction and pinning extremely difficult and open reduction is often necessary. A recent study suggests that these fractures occur in older children, that open reduction is three times more common, and that ulnar nerve injury is six times more common [41].

Complete Physeal Displacement

This variant of the supracondylar fracture occurs exclusively in children under the age of 2 years. Because the capitellar epiphysis is the first to appear at the age of 12 months these fractures can be difficult to diagnose, masquerading either as elbow dislocations or lateral condyle fractures. The fractures are high-energy injuries and child abuse must always be considered as a possible cause. Another recognized cause is birth trauma, and the injury may be misdiagnosed as an obstetric brachial plexus palsy [42].

The key to diagnosis is an index of suspicion. The best investigations to confirm the diagnosis are ultrasound and arthrography. Of these, ultrasound is superior because it can be used in the conscious infant. Arthrography is a useful adjunct to the operative procedure. Because the displacement is at the level of the physis, rather than in the thin metaphysis, where the conventional supracondylar fracture occurs, the fracture may be much more stable after closed reduction. Some authors therefore recommend closed reduction with traction and a cast, while others feel that this fracture should be pinned to prevent later deformity. Just as in the supracondylar fracture, deformity in the plane of the elbow joint remodels well, whereas valgus and varus do not.

Lateral Condyle Fractures

These fractures are the second most common children's elbow fracture to need operative treatment. The fracture is unusual for a child's fracture in that:
(1) The fracture heals slowly.
(2) Late deformity can occur.
(3) Non-union is a recognized complication.

The fracture crosses both the joint line and the physis. It should therefore be regarded as a Salter–Harris IV fracture, whether or not the fracture line transects the bony epiphysis. If the fracture line extends beyond the bony epiphysis of the capitellum toward the middle of the joint, then displacement is likely to be much more extensive and the injury is a fracture dislocation.

The diagnosis is made on plain X-rays. Pitfalls are that the films may be of poor quality and out of plane; the metaphyseal fragment can be very small; and displacement rather subtle. Ultrasound can be a useful aid to diagnosis, and several authors have described arthrography to confirm the diagnosis and decide whether operative stabilization is required [43, 44].

Treatment

Essentially *undisplaced lateral condyle fractures* are likely to have intact articular cartilage medially and therefore will not displace any further. These can be treated by immobilization in a sling with or without a split long arm cast. X-rays during and at the end of treatment should be taken to ensure that there is neither delayed displacement nor non-union.

Displaced fractures are likely to displace further due to the pull of the common extensors of the forearm, and therefore should be stabilized. There is general agreement that these fractures should be stabilized and there are two common techniques.

The first of these is open reduction through a lateral approach (Kocher) and stabilization with two divergent

Fig. 6.9 K-wire fixation of a displaced lateral condyle fracture

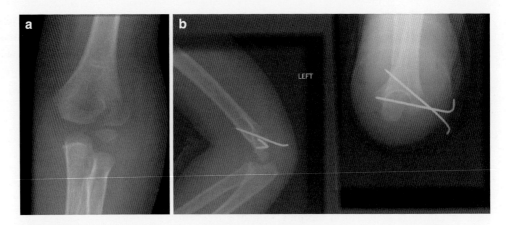

Fig. 6.10 Posterior screw fixation of displaced lateral condyle fracture

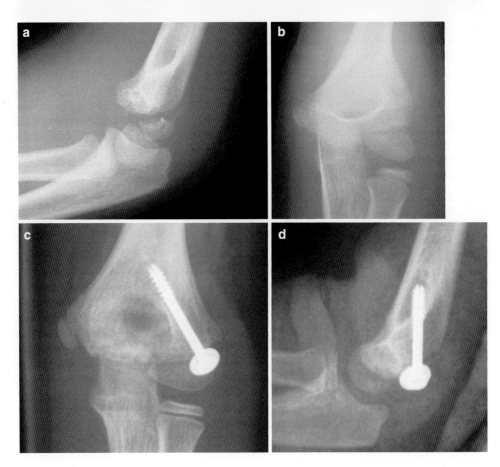

K-wires. Reduction of the joint is observed through an anterior arthrotomy, and no posterior dissection is undertaken in order to protect the blood supply to the fragment. The K-wires are buried under the skin and a long arm cast or a sugar tong splint is applied for immobilization. Healing is generally achieved in 5 weeks. The buried K-wires are removed under general anesthesia in a day clinic; if the wires are not buried they can be removed in the clinic (Fig. 6.9).

Some deformity of the lateral supracondylar ridge has been noted in follow-up studies of these cases [45].The alternative involves screw fixation of the fracture through the metaphyseal fragment [46] (Fig. 6.10). Provided the

common extensor origin is left attached to the fragment it will remain fully vascularized, and the screw can be inserted through the metaphyseal fragment, which is frequently quite large but not well seen from a lateral approach. The advantages of screw fixation are that mobilization can be begun quite early and deformity of the supracondylar ridge is less often seen [47]. The disadvantages are that the screw cannot be used in small children and that the implant removal is a more formal operation.

There is a group of fractures that present rather late. Controversy exists as to at when one should abandon attempts at anatomical reduction. Recent publications

Fig. 6.11 CT of incarcerated medial epicondyle after elbow dislocation and reduction

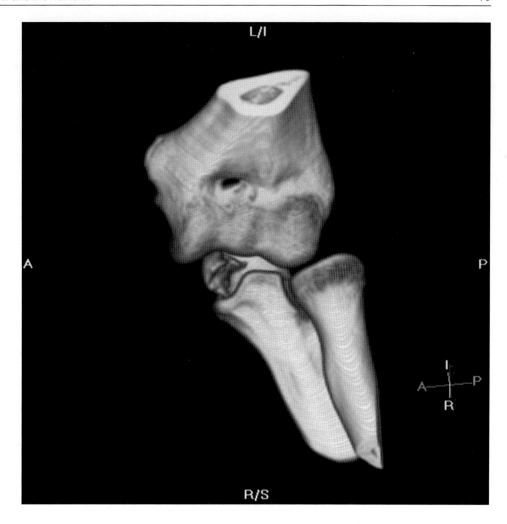

suggest that the window for treatment closes at 6–8 weeks. This seems unnecessarily conservative for a group of fractures that by definition are displaced and slow to heal. Even at 12 weeks the fracture line can be identified in delayed and mal-union and, provided the main soft tissue attachment of the common extensor is left attached, then repositioning is reasonable [48].

Treatment of Late Cases

Conservative treatment of a displaced lateral condyle fracture is usually not successful and leads to non-union. Late diagnosed cases of lateral condyle non-unions are characterized by surprisingly good function in terms of elbow movements. Children present with valgus deformity of the distal humerus and/or with tardy ulnar palsy. Union is achieved by open reduction, autologous bone grafting, pinning by several K-wires, or screw fixation, if the physis is about to terminate growth. Nerve compression often needs ulnar nerve transfer rather than simple decompression.

In very late cases, the objective should be to obtain union of the fracture and prevent further deformity, rather than attempt anatomical reduction which may cause the fragment to lose its blood supply. Having achieved union of the fragment, more proximal osteotomies may be required to achieve the correct alignment of the arm. The variety of different osteotomies described suggests that none is superior and corrective procedures may be accompanied by more residual deformity than operator or parents expect [49, 50].

Fractures of the Medial Epicondyle

Fractures of the medial epicondyle are exclusively associated with dislocations of the elbow joint. Few other injuries produce sufficient force to avulse the epicondyle. Fifty percent of these injuries have a dislocated elbow at the time of presentation. Most of the remainder will have suffered a transient dislocation or subluxation (Fig. 6.11).

The treatment of avulsion fracture of the medial epicondyle is controversial. Undisplaced fractures may be

Fig. 6.12 T-fracture of distal humerus fixed percutaneously

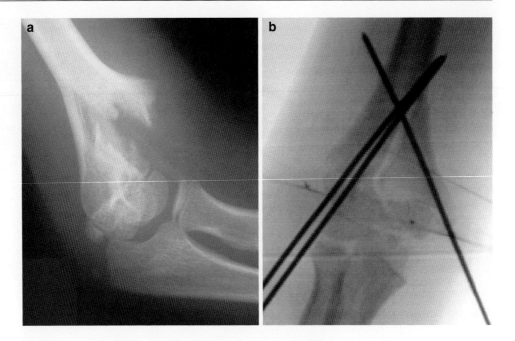

treated non-operatively, but there is little agreement as to what constitutes an undisplaced fracture. The most invasive will only accept 2 mm displacement. About 5–10 mm is commonly accepted, while a long-term follow-up study has suggested that the functional outcome is satisfactory even with 15 mm displacement. Poor results happen: the epicondyle may become stuck down to the medial aspect of the trochlea; sometimes the medial epicondyle becomes entrapped within the joint. This does require intervention, and although closed maneuvers to remove the epicondyle are described, open reduction and fixation are probably superior.

If operation is required, an approach sufficiently large to visualize the ulnar nerve is advisable. In young children two K-wires will be more appropriate to fix a displaced fragment. A long arm cast must be used for 3–5 weeks. If the patient is old enough the medial epicondyle is fixed with a screw as mobilization can then start as soon as the soft tissues have settled down. Mercer Rang recommended fixing these fractures with the patient prone and the affected arm behind the back as this makes reduction easier.

It is important to remember that medial epicondyle avulsions always occur in association with traumatic elbow dislocation and have a relatively high risk of impaired elbow function irrespective of whether they are treated conservatively or operatively. Elbow stiffness should be considered more as a sequel of the ruptured capsule than of the avulsed epicondyle. Parents should be warned about this.

Complete Articular Fractures of the Distal Humerus—T-Fractures

These unusual fractures require reconstitution of the articular surface and suitable re-attachment to the shaft. The treatment chosen depends on the patient's age and the fracture complexity. They usually occur in adolescents who are close to the end of growth, and the fracture patterns resemble those of adults. They should be treated like an adult fracture with precise open reduction and plate fixation. Slightly premature elbow closure will not cause any deformity or length discrepancy. Fractures that occur in the younger age group may have intact articular cartilage with the T being a metaphyseal split only. In that situation treatment should be as for supracondylar fractures although a medial wire is advisable. Preoperative CT scan or arthrography may aid the diagnosis [42]. In those rare cases when a younger child is injured, it may be possible to reduce and hold the fracture with percutaneous wires, thereby avoiding an extensive surgical approach [51] (Fig. 6.12).

References

1. Andersen K, Jensen PO, Lauritzen J. Treatment of clavicular fractures. Figure-of-eight bandage versus a simple sling. Acta Orthop Scand 1987; 58:71–74.
2. Kubiak R, Slongo T. Operative treatment of clavicle fractures in children: a review of 21 years. J Pediatr Orthop 2002; 22:736–739.

3. Al-Qattan MM, Clarke HM, Curtis CG. The prognostic value of concurrent clavicular fractures in newborns with obstetric brachial plexus palsy. J Hand Surg [Br] 1994; 19:729–730.

4. Ogden JA. Distal clavicular physeal injury. Clin Orthop Relat Res 1984; 188:68–73.

5. Waters PM, Bae DS, Kadiyala RK. Short-term outcomes after surgical treatment of traumatic posterior sternoclavicular fracture-dislocations in children and adolescents. J Pediatr Orthop 2003; 23:464–469.

6. Landin LA. Fracture patterns in children. Analysis of 8682 fractures with special reference to incidence, etiology and secular changes in a Swedish urban population, 1950–1979. Acta Orthop Scand Suppl 1983; 3:54

7. Slongo T, Audige L, Clavert JM, Lutz N, Frick S, Hunter J. The AO comprehensive classification of pediatric long-bone fractures: a web-based multicenter agreement study. J Pediatr Orthop 2007; 27:171–180.

8. Broker F, Burbach T. Ultrasonic diagnosis of separation of the proximal humeral epiphysis in the newborn. J Bone Joint Surg (Am) 1990; 72:187–191.

9. Rang M. Children's fractures. 2nd ed. Philadelphia: Lippincott; Philadelphia, Toront; 1983.

10. Chee Y, Agorastides I, Garg N, et al. Treatment of severely displaced proximal humeral fractures in children with elastic stable intramedullary nailing. J Pediatr Orthop B 2006; 15: 45–50.

11. Lucas JC, Mehlman CT, Laor T. The location of the biceps tendon in completely displaced proximal humerus fractures in children: a report of four cases with magnetic resonance imaging and cadaveric correlation. J Pediatr Orthop 2004; 24: 249–253.

12. Dietz H-G, Schmittenbecher PP, Slongo T, Wilkins K. AO Manual of Fracture Management—Elastic Stable Intramedullary Nailing (ESIN) in Children. Stuttgart. New York: Thieme; 2006.

13. Lascombe P. L'embrochage centromédullaire élastique stable Elsevier-Masson 2006; 107–123

14. Worlock P, Stower M, Barbor P. Patterns of fractures in accidental and non-accidental injury in children: a comparative study. Br Med J (Clin Res Ed) 1986; 293(6539):100–102.

15. Shaw BA, Murphy KM, Shaw A, Oppenheim WL, Myracle MR. Humerus shaft fractures in young children: accident or abuse? J Pediatr Orthop 1997; 17:293–297.

16. Loder RT, Feinberg JR. Orthopaedic injuries in children with non-accidental trauma: demographics and incidence from the 2000 kids' inpatient database. J Pediatr Orthop 2007; 27:421–426.

17. Kasser JR, Beaty JH. Supracondylar fractures of the humerus. In: Beaty JH and Kasser JR eds., Rockwood and Wilkins' Fractures in Children. 5th ed. Lippincott: Williams & Wilkins Philadelphia; 2002

18. Gartland JJ. Management of supracondylar fractures of the humerus in children. Surg Gyn Obstet 1959; 109:145–154.

19. Mubarak SJ, Davids J. Closed reduction and percutaneous pinning of the supracondylar fracture in the child. In: Morrey BF, ed. Master Techniques in Orthopaedic Surgery. The Elbow. New York: Raven Press; 1994: 37.

20. Wilkins KE. Supracondylar fractures: what's new? J Pediatr Orthop B 1997; 6:110–116.

21. von Laer L, Gunter SM, Knopf S, Weinberg AM. Supracondylar humerus fracture in childhood—an efficacy study. Results of a multicenter study by the Pediatric Traumatology Section of the German Society of Trauma Surgery—II: Costs and effectiveness of the treatment. Unfallchirurg 2002; 105:217–223

22. Skaggs DL, Sankar WN, Albrektson J, Vaishnav S, Choi PD, Kay RM. How safe is the operative treatment of Gartland type 2

23. Clavert JM, Lecerf C, Mathieu JC, Buck P. Retention in flexion of supracondylar fracture of the humerus in children. Comments apropos of the treatment of 120 displaced fractures. Rev Chir Orthop Reparatrice Appar Mot 1984; 70:109–116

24. Chen RS, Liu CB, Lin XS, Feng XM, Zhu JM, Ye FQ. Supracondylar extension fracture of the humerus in children. Manipulative reduction, immobilisation and fixation using a U-shaped plaster slab with the elbow in full extension. J Bone Joint Surg Br 2001; 83:883–887.

25. Gadgil A, Hayhurst C, Maffulli N, Dwyer JS. Elevated, straight-arm traction for supracondylar fractures of the humerus in children. J Bone Joint Surg Br 2005; 87:82–87.

26. Badhe NP, Howard PW. Olecranon screw traction for displaced supracondylar fractures of the humerus in children. Injury 1998; 29:457–460.

27. Skaggs DL, Hale JM, Bassett J, Kaminsky C, Kay RM, Tolo VT. Operative treatment of supracondylar fractures of the humerus in children. The consequences of pin placement. J Bone Joint Surg Am 2001; 83:735–740.

28. Skaggs DL, Cluck MW, Mostofi A, Flynn JM, Kay RM. Lateral-entry pin fixation in the management of supracondylar fractures in children. J Bone Joint Surg Am 2004; 86:702–707.

29. Reynolds RA, Jackson H. Concept of treatment in supracondylar humeral fractures. Injury 2005; 36(Suppl 1):A51–56.

30. Zenios M, Ramachandran M, Milne B, Little D, Smith N. Intraoperative stability testing of lateral-entry pin fixation of pediatric supracondylar humeral fractures. J Pediatr Orthop 2007; 27:695–702.

31. Zionts LE, McKellop HA, Hathaway R. Torsional strength of pin configurations used to fix supracondylar fractures of the humerus in children. J Bone Joint Surg Am 1994; 76:253–256.

32. Eberhardt O, Fernandez F, Ilchmann T, Parsch K. Cross pinning of supracondylar fractures from a lateral approach. Stabilization achieved with safety. J Child Orthop 2007; 1:127–133

33. Prevot J, Lascombes P, Metaizeau JP, Blanquart D. Supracondylar fractures of the humerus in children: treatment by downward nailing. Rev Chir Orthop Reparatrice Appar Mot 1990; 76:191–197.

34. Slongo T, Jakob RP. The small AO external fixator in paediatric orthopaedics and trauma. Injury 1994; 25(Suppl 4):S-D77–84.

35. Mubarak SJ, Carroll NC. Volkmann's contracture in children: aetiology and prevention. J Bone Joint Surg Br 1979; 61: 285–293.

36. Garbuz DS, Leitch K, Wright JG. The treatment of supracondylar fractures in children with an absent radial pulse. J Pediatr Orthop 1996; 16:594–596.

37. Lewis J, Monk J, Chandratreya A, Hunter J. Changing the management from olecranon screw traction to percutaneous wiring for displaced supracondylar fractures of the humerus in children. A justified decision? Eur J Trauma Emerg Surg 2007; 33: 256–261.

38. Luria S, Sucar A, Eylon S, et al. Vascular complications of supracondylar humeral fractures in children. J Pediatr Orthop B 2007; 16:133–143.

39. Lewis HG, Morrison CM, Kennedy PT, Herbert KJ. Arterial reconstruction using the basilic vein from the zone of injury in pediatric supracondylar humeral fractures: a clinical and radiological series. Plast Reconstr Surg 2003; 111:1159–1163; discussion 1164–1156.

40. Holden C. The pathology and prevention of Volkmann's ischaemic contracture. J Bone Joint Surg Br 1979; 61:296—300.

41. Mahan ST, May CD, Kocher MS. Operative management of displaced flexion supracondylar humerus fractures in children. J Pediatr Orthop 2007; 27:551–556.

supracondylar humerus fractures in children? J Pediatr Orthop 2008; 28:139–141.

42. Blane CE, Kling TF, Jr., Andrews JC, DiPietro MA, Hensinger RN. Arthrography in the posttraumatic elbow in children Am J Roentgenol 1984; 143:17–21.

43. Marzo JM, d'Amato C, Strong M, Gillespie R. Usefulness and accuracy of arthrography in management of lateral humeral condyle fractures in children. J Pediatr Orthop 1990; 10:317–321.

44. Mintzer CM, Waters PM, Brown DJ, Kasser JR. Percutaneous pinning in the treatment of displaced lateral condyle fractures. J Pediatr Orthop 1994; 14:462–465.

45. Thomas DP, Howard AW, Cole WG, Hedden DM. Three weeks of Kirschner wire fixation for displaced lateral condylar fractures of the humerus in children. J Pediatr Orthop 2001; 21:565–569.

46. Mohan N, Hunter JB, Colton CL. The posterolateral approach to the distal humerus for open reduction and internal fixation of fractures of the lateral condyle in children. J Bone Joint Surg Br 2000; 82:643–645.

47. Hasler CC, von Laer L. Prevention of growth disturbances after fractures of the lateral humeral condyle in children. J Pediatr Orthop B 2001; 10:123–130.

48. Wattenbarger JM, Gerardi J, Johnston CE. Late open reduction internal fixation of lateral condyle fractures. J Pediatr Orthop 2002; 22:394–398.

49. Tien YC, Chen JC, Fu YC, Chih TT, Hunag PJ, Wang GJ. Supracondylar dome osteotomy for cubitus valgus deformity associated with a lateral condylar nonunion in children. J Bone Joint Surg Amul 2005; 87:1456–1463.

50. Kim HS, Jahng JS, Han DY, Park HW, Kang HJ, Chun CH. Modified step-cut osteotomy of the humerus. J Pediatr Orthop B 1998; 7:162–166.

51. Ruiz AL, Kealey WD, Cowie HG. Percutaneous pin fixation of intercondylar fractures in young children. J Pediatr Orthop B 2001; 10:211–213.

Chapter 7

Fractures of the Elbow and Forearm

James B. Hunter and Klaus Parsch

Radial Neck

The radial head develops a secondary ossification center, the second to appear at the elbow during childhood, by the age of 3 years or slightly afterward. The radial head is therefore largely made of cartilage and intraarticular fractures are rare. In comparison, the radial neck is commonly fractured, either as a metaphyseal fracture, or as a growth plate injury (Salter Harris I or II). The typical mechanism of injury is a fall on the extended arm with the forces resolving to produce elbow extension and valgus. Radial neck fractures also occur in combination with elbow dislocation. It is vital to diagnose these since the reduction maneuver may otherwise result in full displacement of a previously undisplaced fracture.

The classification of radial neck fractures is somewhat unsatisfactory. Judet's classification has been most widely used but has proved unreliable [1]. Classifications have either concentrated upon the degree of angulation of the fracture, or on the amount of displacement. The key anatomical feature that determines functional outcome is the relationship between the radial head and the annular ligament. This is much more affected by displacement than by angulation, such that quite marked angulation can be accepted, while almost any displacement will need correction. The AO classification distinguishes between metaphyseal and growth plate injuries and uses a simple three-group system for severity (Fig. 7.1):

 I. fracture with no angulation and no displacement
 II. fracture with angulation and displacement, up to 50% of the bone diameter
 III. fracture displaced more than 50% of the bone diameter

J.B. Hunter (✉)
Departments of Trauma and Orthopaedics, Nottingham University Hospital, Nottingham, UK

Treatment

Many angulated radial neck fractures require no treatment other than early mobilization. All authors would accept 30° of angulation, and some have suggested that more (up to 50°) can be treated conservatively provided there is no displacement [2].

Displaced fractures need to be reduced but closed reduction can be difficult, because of the problems of reducing the distal fragment to the proximal fragment. Manipulation involves the application a valgus force to the elbow and pressure over the radial head to reduce it. This maneuver needs to be accompanied by rotation of the forearm, but is frequently unsuccessful. Semi-closed methods, using a large diameter percutaneous K-wire, are frequently used. We prefer to use the flat end of a 3 mm wire to push against the radial head directly, rather than using the sharp end in the fracture gap, which can endanger the posterior interosseous nerve or the blood supply [3]. This method is frequently used in conjunction with the technique of Metaizeau in which an intramedullary elastic nail or K-wire is used both to reduce the fracture and to stabilize it, allowing early mobilization [4]. This is now the most popular method throughout Europe (Fig. 7.2).

The key steps are shown in Fig. 7.3:

1. Partially reduce using manipulation or K-wire.
2. Visualize maximum displacement under the image intensifier.
3. Direct bent nail into the head, disimpacting the fracture.
4. Rotate the nail to reduce the fracture.

Open reduction is only rarely required if the combination of the above techniques has failed. Generally, this only occurs if the radial head is fully displaced and lying parallel to the shaft. In some circumstances, the radial head may be flipped over, such that the articular surface is facing the fracture site. This occurs most frequently when radial neck fracture is associated with elbow dislocation, the

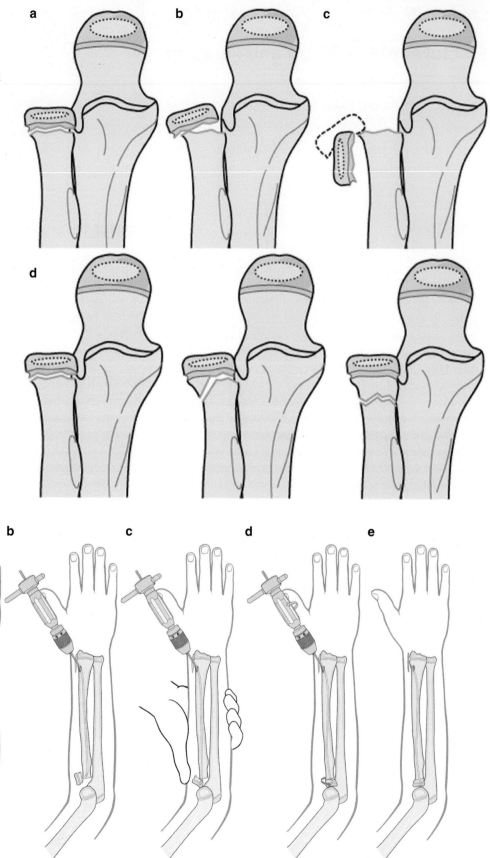

Fig. 7.1 Classification of radial neck fractures. (**a**) Undisplaced fracture. (**b**) Fracture displaced up to 50% neck diameter. (**c**) Fracture displaced more than 50%. (**d**) Fracture can be physeal (Salter–Harris I or II) or metaphyseal. From: Slongo T, Audigé L, AO Classification Group. AO Pediatric Comprehensive Classification of Long Bone Fractures (PCCF). Davos, Switzerland: AO Publishing; 2007. Used with permission

Fig. 7.2 Metaizeau technique for reduction and stabilization of radial neck fractures. From: Dietz H-G, Schmittenbecher P, Slongo T. AO Manual of Fracture Management: Elastic Stable Intramedullary nailing (ESIN) in Children. Davos, Switzerland: AO Publishing; 2006. Used with permission

Fig. 7.3 Radiographs of radial neck fracture treated by Metaizeau technique

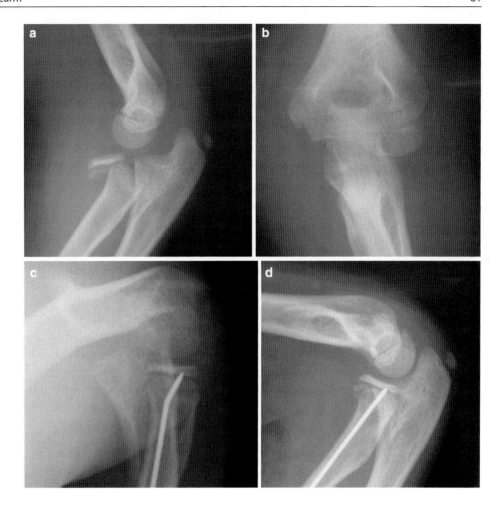

inversion occurring during attempted reduction. The surgical approach is determined by the position of the radial head, and sometimes an anterior approach (Henry) is appropriate. A sigmoid, transverse incision is much more cosmetic than a longitudinal incision crossing the elbow. If a lateral approach is used, then great care must be taken to preserve the periosteal sleeve that is attached to the radial head. This contains the blood supply so that an over-invasive open reduction is associated with avascular necrosis of the radial head and non-union of the fracture. Intramedullary stabilization is still preferable, even after open reduction, to allow forearm rotation during healing.

Olecranon Fractures

True olecranon fractures are relatively rare in children, especially when one considers how often they graze their elbows. This is because the olecranon is largely composed of cartilage during childhood. The proximal apophysis appears at around the age of 9 years, and fuses to the ulnar shaft at the end of the growth spurt after becoming bipartite and

enlarging. At this stage, it is somewhat vulnerable both to fracture and misdiagnosis. Olecranon fractures can be sleeve fractures in which a large portion of articular cartilage is contained within a fragment that appears to be extra-articular. Displaced olecranon fractures should be explored, reduced, and stabilized accurately. Tension band wiring, as used in adult practice, is the technique of choice; wires of appropriate diameter for the size of the child should be used, and the elbow mobilized early (Fig. 7.4).

More complex fractures of the proximal ulna are frequently associated with Monteggia injuries and are considered below.

Fractures of the Radial and Ulnar Shafts

These are the most common diaphyseal injuries of childhood. Generally, the mechanism is a simple fall, frequently from a modest height, such as a gate or playground equipment. All types of childhood diaphyseal injury are seen, often in combination. Thus a complete fracture of the radius may be seen with plastic deformity of the ulna, and the

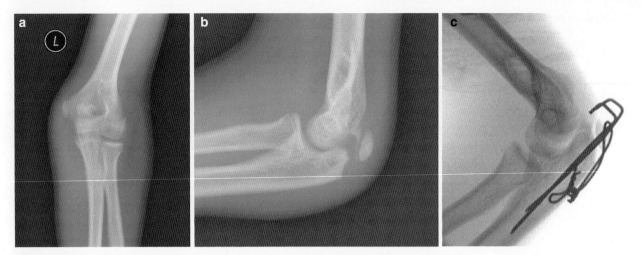

Fig. 7.4 Olecranon fracture treated by tension band wiring, although apparently extra-articular a large sleeve of articular cartilage was attached to the fragment

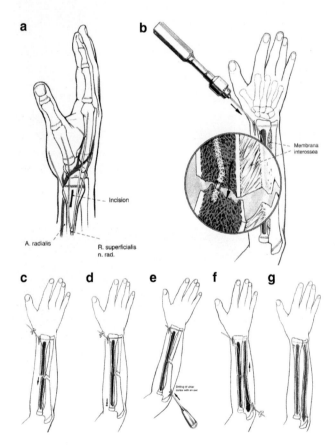

Fig. 7.5 Intramedullary elastic pinning with blunt K-wire From Parsch K. Morote pinning Orthopaedic Traumatologic operations 1992 Copyright © Urban and Vogel. Reproduced with permission **a**) Entry point for radial elastic wire. **b**) blunt prebent K-wire passes the fracture by rotating back and forth reducing the fracture. **c**) Radial wire is moving past the fracture. **d**) Radial wire has reached the radial neck, aligning the radial fracture. **e**) An awl opens the medullary canal of the proximal ulna distal to the olecranon. **f**) The ulnar wire is pushed past the ulna fracture by rotatory movements. **g**) The wire ends are cut 10 mm distal the entry point and bent 150 degrees and impacted into the periostium. The skin is closed

different behavior of these fracture types may affect management. The vast majority of these fractures are incomplete and undisplaced, although angulated sufficiently to require active management. The relationship between the radius and ulna must be accurately maintained to preserve forearm rotation. In adult practice, anatomical reduction is required for pronation and supination; in children this is not the case, because the periosteal sleeve and the interosseous membrane are generally intact, and because some remodeling will take place, albeit less than in the metaphyses.

Conservative Treatment

Angulation is the main cause of lost forearm rotation. Every 10° of angulation in the midshaft will lead to a loss of 20° of total forearm rotation (180°) [5, 6]. If forearm rotation is blocked, then remodeling will not occur satisfactorily. Therefore, 10° of angulation developing during follow-up is acceptable, but more is not. If angulation does develop, then it should be corrected, either by re-manipulation or by wedging of the cast, which can be achieved in the clinic under appropriate analgesia.

Displacement of forearm shaft fractures is important, because of the effect it has upon angulation. In younger children (8 years and under), bayonet apposition of the radius and the shaft is acceptable provided both bones have displaced in the same direction and the interosseous distance is maintained. In this situation, healing occurs quickly and rotation can resume before any permanent stiffness develops. If one fracture is reduced and the other displaced, the situation is unstable and likely to tip into angulation. If managed conservatively, the cast must be carefully molded into an oval shape to spread the interosseous membrane (as it must for all radial and ulnar fractures), and careful, weekly follow-up instituted as angulation may occur quite late.

Rotation at the fracture site is classically judged using the method of Evans, assessing the appearance of the bicipital tuberosity and comparing it with the appearance of the distal radius [7]. Use of this method has led to the recommendation that 30° of rotational mismatch can be accepted in the management of forearm shaft fractures [8]. From first principles this seems unlikely, particularly as Evans's method can be very difficult to use in the young child. Reductions in which there is obvious rotational mismatch of the diameter of the radius and ulna are unlikely to be correct, and re-reduction is recommended [6].

The main debate in the treatment of these fractures in children concerns how much angulation can be accepted in the expectation of remodeling, and how much morbidity actually results from residual angulation. Papers from the last decades of the 20th century suggested that there was little loss of movement as a result of conservative management of these fractures [6, 8]. A more critical analysis from Central Europe found a relatively high rate of malunion, and loss of motion associated with it [9]. Typical results were a re-reduction rate of 10%, visible residual deformity at follow-up in more than 10%, and a greater than 20° loss of forearm rotation in 7%. Some papers found loss of rotation to be greatest when the fractures were at the same level, while others found loss of function to be worst with proximal radial fractures [10]. Therefore, when treated conservatively forearm fractures require a relatively long period of immobilization and very careful follow-up.

Surgical Treatment

The combination of a moderately high risk of less than perfect results, the need for multiple visits, and the availability of a less invasive method of osteosynthesis (elastic stable intramedullary nailing, or ESIN) has led to more of these fractures being treated operatively in the last 25 years. Good results have been reported using both formal elastic nails and K-wires inserted by the same technique (Fig. 7.6) [11–14]. Our policy is to use elastic nails primarily for all fully displaced (off-ended) diaphyseal fractures of the radius and ulna, except for children under 6 years of age. The reason for this seemingly aggressive policy is that closed nailing is much more likely if the nails are used at the first operation rather than at any later procedure. The learning curve for nailing is such that in the third year of practice, 85% of these cases can be dealt with by closed nailing [14]. The infection rate is minimal and the main complication seems to be a slight increase in the incidence of compartment syndrome [15]. This probably results because any open reduction is normally done through a minimal approach in the line of the Thompson incision, insufficient to decompress the volar forearm compartments; secondly, elastic nails prevent loss of reduction by shortening which would normally lead to a reduction in compartment pressure.

The technique for intramedullary nailing of the radius and ulna is relatively simple [3, 13, 14] (Fig. 7.7). The conventional entry points in the distal radial metaphysis are either at the base of the radial styloid or Lister's tubercle. If the

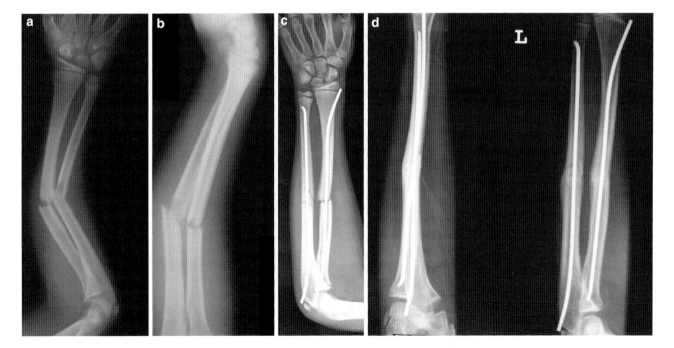

Fig. 7.6 **a**)–**c**) Intramedullary pinning of mid-shaft forearm fracture. **d**) follow-up at 3 months before pin removal

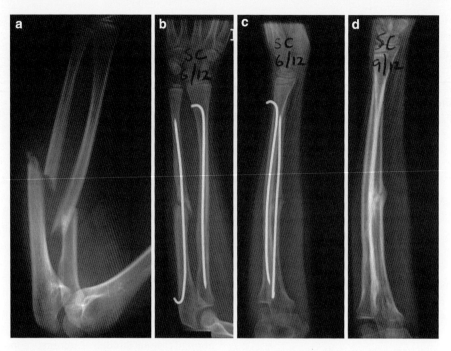

Fig. 7.7 **a**) dislocated mid-shaft forearm fracture in a 10-year-old boy. **b**) after 2 months low healing tendancy. **c**) Five months after fracture solid healing. **d**)The stainless steel wires have been removed

former is chosen, care must be taken to avoid the superficial branches of the radial nerve. If the latter is chosen it is the extensor tendons that are at risk. Damage to these can be avoided by an adequate incision to visualize the insertion point and by leaving the nail long so that the cut end is not in the same plane as the tendons but in the subcutaneous fat. If Kirschner wires are used they are bent over to form a "pig's tail" thus avoiding irritation to the soft tissues. The ulna is conventionally pinned from the lateral side of the proximal metaphysis, which is easily and safely accessible. This can be a little awkward with positioning and image intensification, so a start point in the distal metaphysis has been described [3]. The radial nail should be contoured to recreate the bow of the radius thus stretching the interosseous membrane. The ulnar nail is generally straight, or gently contoured to keep the ulna straight, preventing it from collapsing toward the radius.

The aftercare of fractures that have been treated by elastic nailing is to mobilize them early. No cast is required. A bandage and a broad arm sling for a few days are all that is required. Elbow, forearm, and wrist movements should be commenced as soon as symptoms permit.

Forearm shaft fractures are relatively slow to heal when compared to other paediatric fractures. Generally, 6 weeks in a cast is required for fractures that have been manipulated. Elastic nailing of these fractures is associated with slower healing, particularly if open reduction has been required [16]. Another factor implicated in slow healing may be the use of nails that are too stiff, either because they are too broad or made of steel. Nail or K-wire diameters should be between 1.6 and 1.8 mm if they are made of stainless steel and 1.5 or 2 mm if they are made of titanium, depending upon age (Fig. 7.8).

The Nancy group recommend that the nails be left in situ for 6 months before retrieval [13, 17]. Retrieval is recommended in all cases. If secondary fractures occur with nails still in place these can either be bent straight and immobilized in a cast or, more usually, be replaced by new nails.

Galeazzi Fractures

Galeazzi fractures of the radius with dislocation of the distal radio-ulnar joint are less common than isolated fractures of the radius in children. They generally occur in adolescence shortly before maturity. This is because the ligaments and capsule of the joint are extremely strong. The principle of management is accurate reduction of the radius to allow healing of the joint capsule. The method of stabilization of the radius will depend upon the level of the fracture: diaphysis—elastic nail; junction of metaphysis and diaphysis—plate; distal radius—K-wires. Immobilization in pronation is recommended, but this should not be too prolonged as ligaments and capsule require movement for effective healing.

Fig. 7.8 Mid-shaft fracture in 9-year old boy treated with intramedullary Morote wires

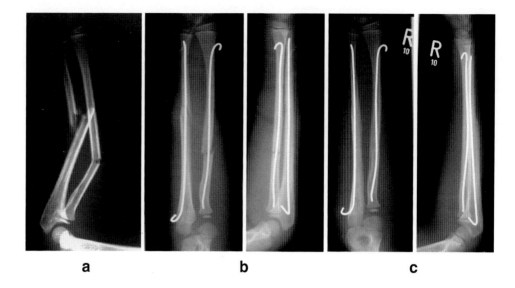

a   b   c

Monteggia Fracture Dislocation

In the early 19th century Giovanni Battista Monteggia, Professor of Surgery in Milan, described the clinical picture of a fracture of the proximal ulna in a young girl which, after healing, was followed by a hard and ugly prominence on the anterior surface of the elbow identified as a "jumping radius." [18].

The classification is detailed in Fig. 7.9. Bado from Montevideo defined the Monteggia lesion as an association of a radial head dislocation or fracture with a fracture of the middle or proximal ulna and described four types: [19]

- Type I: anterior dislocation of the radial head in combination with an anteriorly angulated, mid-shaft ulnar fracture. About 70% of Monteggia injuries belong to this group.
- Type II: posterior dislocation of the radial head in combination with a very proximal metaphyseal fracture of the ulna, angulated posteriorly. Bado type II lesions are rare and are more common in adults than in children, where they have a frequency of only 3% [20].
- Type III: the radial head is dislocated antero-laterally in association with a fracture of the ulnar metaphysis. This type accounts for 23% of these fractures in children [20].

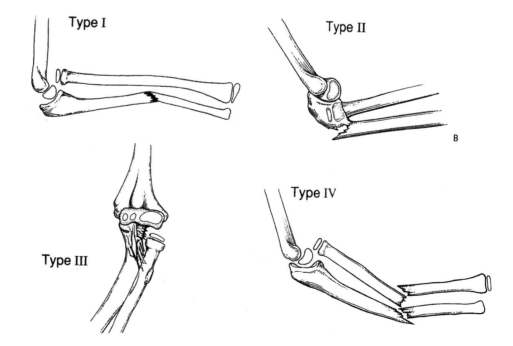

Fig. 7.9 Bado classification of Monteggia lesions. Reproduced with permission from Stanley EA, de la Garza JF. Monteggia fracture dislocations in children. Part III. In Rockwood And Wilkins' Fractures in children. 5th edition. Editors: JH Beaty and JR Kasser Philadelphia PA, Lippicott Williams & Wilkins 2001

- Type IV: an anterior dislocation of the radial head in combination with a fracture of both radius and ulna at the same level. This combination is rare, only 1% of the total [21, 22].

Monteggia Equivalent (Variant) Injuries

In addition to the classic Monteggia lesion, Bado classified certain injuries as Monteggia equivalents:

Type I equivalent (variant) is an isolated anterior dislocation of the radial head with a minimal plastic deformation of the ulna which might not be visible radiographically. The pulled elbow with radial head subluxation under the annular ligament is also classified as a Monteggia equivalent. Another type I equivalent is the combination of a fracture of the ulnar diaphysis with fracture of the radial neck.

Type II equivalent is an epiphyseal fracture of the radial head or radial neck.

Type III and type IV Monteggia equivalents are extremely rare.

Letts et al. [23] based their classification of Monteggia fractures upon both the direction of radial head displacement and the type of ulnar fracture. Bado type I lesions were subdivided into three groups:

Letts type A is a bowing fracture of the ulna with anterior dislocation of the radial head. Type B shows a greenstick fracture of the ulna, while type C has a complete ulnar fracture. Letts type D corresponds to Bado type II, while type E corresponds to Bado type III.

Mechanism of Injury

Three different mechanisms have been considered to cause Monteggia type I lesion:

- *The direct blow theory* is attributable to Monteggia himself in his description of the girl who was the index case [18]. A direct blow to the forearm can cause a transverse fracture of the ulna and anterior dislocation of the radial head.
- *The hyperpronation theory* has been favored by Bado [19]. The child falls on the pronated forearm in extension, fracturing the ulna and dislocating the radial head during further pronation in extension.
- *The hyperextension theory* described by Tompkins recognized the forward momentum caused by a fall on the outstretched hand, forcing the elbow into extension. Sudden biceps contraction forcibly dislocates the radial head. The forward momentum then fractures the ulna because the radius is no longer the weight transmitting

bone of the forearm. This theory combines dynamic and static forces [24].

Anatomy

The *annular ligament* provides stability for the radial head and its position within the radial notch of the ulna. In children the radial head pulls out of the intact annular ligament, while in adults the injury tears the ligament. This is one of the main reasons that the Monteggia lesion is more benign in children than in adults [25]. The *quadrate ligament* connecting the radial neck to the proximal ulna adds stability. Distal to the insertion of the biceps tendon the oblique ligament and the interosseous membrane tighten during supination of the radius.

The biceps muscle inserting into the radial tuberosity plays an important role in the pathomechanics of the Monteggia lesion. The posterior interosseous nerve also has a close anatomical relationship to the proximal radius such that acute anterior or lateral dislocation of the radius may cause paresis of this nerve. Recovery of function is usually complete in a few weeks.

Clinical Findings

Considerable swelling around the elbow and severe pain characterize the injury. The child cannot move the elbow in either flexion and extension or pronation and supination. As the swelling subsides a bump may be palpated in the cubital fossa, caused by the radial head.

Radiographic Findings

As in any forearm and elbow injury anteroposterior (AP) and lateral radiographs must always include the neighboring joints. Besides the ulnar fracture or bowing, the relationship of the radial head to the capitellum must be checked. On the AP view the radial head may look normally positioned but on the lateral view a line drawn through the center of the radial head and neck ceases to extend directly through the center of the capitellum [26]. It must be stressed that in suspected Monteggia lesion the radiocapitellar relationship must be very carefully assessed [27].

Treatment of Type I Lesions

Almost all acute type I Monteggia fractures can be treated conservatively; however, many benefit from operative ulnar stabilization. Conservative treatment entails three steps: reduction of the ulna, reduction of the radial head, and immobilization in a well-molded long arm cast.

Reduction of the ulna is achieved by longitudinal traction and manual pressure over the apex of the angular deformity. With greenstick fractures and plastic deformation of the ulna, reduction is equally necessary in order to gain length, allow for reduction of the radial head, and prevent loss of reduction. When the radius is intact it can be difficult to over reduce the plastically deformed ulna past its yield point, so the ulna may need to be osteotomized percutaneously by a drill and chisel technique.

Reduction of the radial head is possible only after restoration of the length and proper alignment of the ulna. The radial head can be located by a simple elbow flexion maneuver.

A well-molded long arm plaster or splint is needed in flexion of 110° in order to reduce the dislocating force of the biceps muscle. Repeated radiographic reviews are necessary to ensure that ulnar alignment and reduction of the radial head is preserved [28]. This approach works well with greenstick fractures but can be a problem in primarily unstable ulna fractures which may later develop malalignment of the ulnar fracture followed by redislocation or subluxation of the radial head.

In the past, unstable ulnar fractures have been fixed by plates [29–31], but intramedullary devices have a major advantage as pins or wires can be introduced with minimal invasiveness. There is a considerable advantage in stabilizing the fracture of the ulna with an intramedullary device under the same anesthetic [14]. The insertion of a K- wire or flexible nail is similar to the treatment of forearm shaft fractures (Fig. 7.10).

In Monteggia equivalent lesions, combining an ulnar fracture with a displaced fracture of the radial neck, the ulna fracture must be reduced and percutaneously pinned. The radial neck and head is then reduced according to the Metaizeau technique (Fig. 7.11).

Treatment of Type II Lesions

This fracture is more common in adults than in children, especially in those with osteoporosis after long-term therapy with corticosteroids [32]. Closed reduction of the ulnar fracture is usually possible by applying longitudinal traction with the elbow held at 60° of flexion. The radial head will reduce spontaneously or by applying local pressure against the posterior aspect of the elbow. If the fracture of the ulna is stable, immobilization in a long arm cast either in full extension or 80° of flexion is ensured for 4–6 weeks until the fracture has healed. In case of instability of the proximal ulna and the risk of repeated posterior dislocation, retrograde pinning is advised, or plate fixation, as in the adult.

Treatment of Type III Lesions

After the correct diagnosis is established, nonoperative treatment is advised and is effective in most cases. A valgus stress corrects the varus deformity of the metaphyseal fracture of the ulna. The radial head will slip back into its correct position during the same maneuver. Reduction of the fracture and of the radial head is monitored radiographically. When the ulna is stable after reduction and the radial head is well aligned, immobilization for 4 weeks in a long arm cast is necessary. If conservative treatment has failed, open reduction and internal fixation are necessary, possibly with repair of the annular ligament. The reduced ulna is either plated or secured by K-wires. A molded long arm cast with the elbow flexed is applied until union. Radiographs must confirm the reduced position of the radial head throughout the healing period.

Treatment of Type IV Lesions

Intramedullary stabilization with blunt K-wires or thin titanium nails is the treatment of choice [12, 14, 17]. After alignment of both ulna and radius the radial head will usually stay reduced. If the child is seen without delay closed reduction and percutaneous pinning are possible.

In delayed cases and larger adolescents open reduction may be necessary. The radius is internally fixed, the radiocapitellar relationship restored, and the ulna plated.

Differential Diagnosis—Congenital Dislocation of the Radial Head

If the radiocapitellar relationship is abnormal, congenital dislocation, with or without radio-ulnar synostosis, should be considered. Posterior radial head displacement can be confused with a Bado type II lesion. Congenital dislocations are often diagnosed quite late, when the child has developed restriction of forearm rotation. The extension deficit may be overlooked for years. True congenital dislocations are usually bilateral and seen in various syndromes like Larsen's or Ehlers–Danlos. Surgery to reduce the congenital dislocation of radial head is not advised; it is unlikely to produce a better range of motion because the radio-ulnar joint is incongruous.

Delayed Diagnosis of Monteggia Lesions

Monteggia lesions, especially the type I, may occur with only ulnar bowing or a greenstick fracture in the midshaft. If careful radiographic examination is omitted persistent dislocation

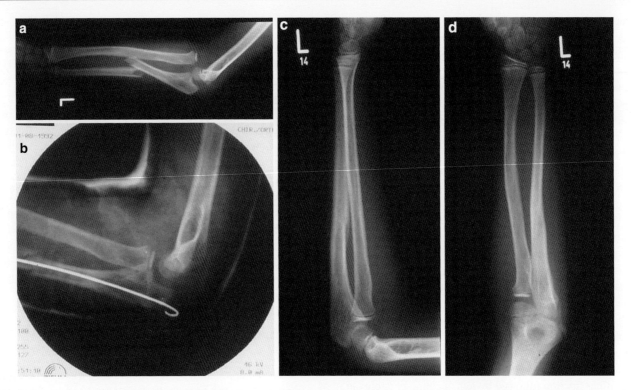

Fig. 7.10 **a**) Type I Monteggia fracture. **b**) Closed reduction of the ulna, closed reduction of the radial head, and stabilization of the ulna by intramedullary K-wire. **c**) and **d**) outcome 6 months after fracture dislocation

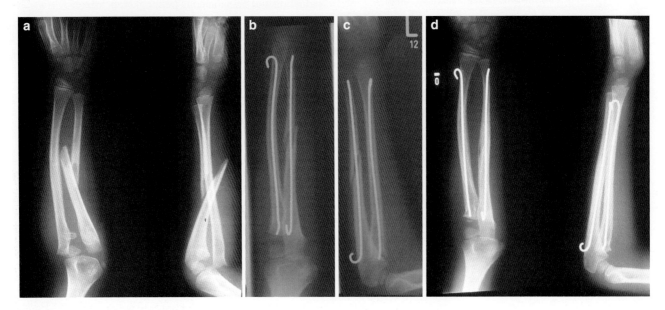

Fig. 7.11 Monteggia variant with displaced fracture of radial neck rather than dislocation. Closed reduction of the ulna and stabilization by intramedullary K-wire, closed reduction and stabilization of dislocated radial neck in the Metaizeau technique (see Fig. 7.3)

may be diagnosed at a later stage, manifest with a fullness in the lateral cubital fossa [33].

If the initial radiographic examinations do not include the elbow joint, most importantly a true lateral view, the dislocation of the radial head will be missed. Children presenting with persistent dislocation of the radial head usually present with insufficient previous radiographs.

Initially, an untreated Monteggia lesion with established radial head displacement is painless and movements are little restricted. In long-standing cases there is restricted motion, both pronation and supination and flexion (caused by impingement of the dislocated radial head). Pain, instability, degenerative joint disease, and late neuropathy may follow [25]. It is unclear how long after injury it is appropriate to attempt correction. Surgical reduction as late as 6 years after the injury has been reported [34].

Treatment of Persistent Dislocation of The Radial Head

Reduction of the Radial Head with Annular Ligament Reconstruction

Conservative methods have no chance of providing a stable radio-humeral joint. Although the annular ligament is not torn during the initial lesion, secondary atrophy occurs with time. Annular ligament reconstructions include reefing [25] or use of a strip of biceps tendon, triceps brachii tendon, or the lacertus fibrosus [35]. We have for many years used a strip taken from fascia lata. To support annular ligament reconstructions a transcapitellar K-wire has been recommended during the initial phase, thus keeping the radial head in the reduced position [33, 34]. Wire breakage and difficulty in implant retrieval are definite risks so a temporary, stabilizing oblique K-wire is safer, augmenting the use of a well-molded, long arm cast.

Osteotomy of The Ulna

An ulnar osteotomy is indicated if there is residual ulnar angulation on the lateral radiograph since radial head reduction will otherwise fail. Corrective osteotomy of the ulna, with or without lengthening, is then secured with a plate [36–39]. Combining this with open reduction and reconstruction of the annular ligament ensures more stability but bears a risk of loss of some pronation (Fig. 7.12). Closed or open reduction by gradual lengthening and angulation using an external fixator has also been suggested for the missed, chronic anterior dislocation of the radial head [40, 41].

Reconstructive surgery is fraught with complications, hence the debate about how late it can be undertaken. Residual radiocapitellar dislocation or subluxation, ulnar nerve palsy, heterotopic ossification, and fibrous synostosis with loss of pronation and supination may complicate the procedure [20, 42].

Summary

Paediatric Monteggia fracture-dislocations and Monteggia variants will do well after conservative treatment by closed reduction if recognized acutely. Fixation of the ulna reduces the risk of secondary malunion and redislocation of the radial head if there is concern about the durability of reduction. Late diagnosis is all too common, partly because the injury may be considered relatively trivial at presentation, but also because diagnostically important radiographs are not requested. The surgical treatment of a long-standing dislocation of the radial head is technically difficult. Angular and lengthening osteotomy of the ulna, with or without reconstruction of the annular ligament, leads to satisfactory results in most cases.

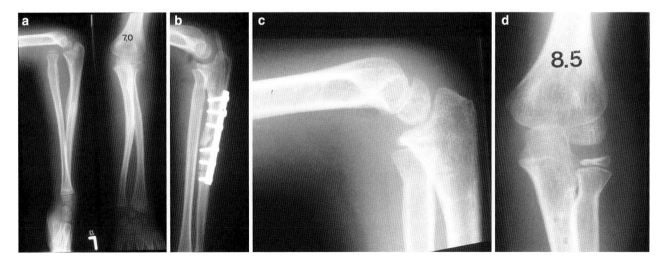

Fig. 7.12 Neglected Monteggia fracture treated by ulnar lengthening and flexion osteotomy, relocation of radial head, and reconstruction of the annular ligament using a fascia lata strip

References

1. Slongo T, Audige L, Clavert JM, Lutz N, Frick S, Hunter J. The AO comprehensive classification of pediatric long-bone fractures: a web-based multicenter agreement study. J Pediatr Orthop 2007; 27(2):171–180.

2. Vocke-Hell AK, von Laer L. Displaced fractures of the radial neck in children: long term results and prognosis with conservative treatment. J Pediatr Orthop Br 1997; 7(3):217–222.

3. Dietz H-G, Schmittenbecher PP, Slongo T, Wilkins K. AO Manual of Fracture Management—Elastic Stable Intramedullary Nailing (ESIN) in Children. Stuttgart, New York: Thieme; 2006.

4. Metaizeau JP, Lascombes P, Lemelle JL, et al. Reduction and fixation of displaced radial neck fractures by closed intramedullary pinning. J Pediatr Orthop 1993; 13(3):355–360.

5. Roberts JA. Angulation of the radius in children's fractures. J Bone Joint Surg Br 1986; 68(5):751–754.

6. Fuller DJ, McCullough CJ. Malunited fractures of the forearm in children. J Bone Joint Surg Br 1982; 64(3):364–367.

7. Evans EM. Fractures of the radius and ulna. J Bone Joint Surg Br 1951; 33:548–561.

8. Price CT, Scott DS, Kurzner ME, Flynn JC. Malunited forearm fractures in children. J Pediatr Orthop 1990; 10(6):705–712.

9. Schmittenbecher PP, Dietz HG, Uhl S. [Late results of forearm fractures in childhood]. Unfallchirurg 1991; 94(4):186–190.

10. Holdsworth BJ, Sloan JP. Proximal forearm fractures in children: residual disability. Injury 1982; 14(2):174–179.

11. Perez-Sicilia J, Morote Jurado J, Corbacho Girones J. Osteosyntesis percutánea en fracturas diafisarias de antebrazo en ninos y adolescentes. Rev Esp Cir Ost 1977; 12:321–334.

12. Verstreken L, Delronge G, Lamoureux J. Shaft forearm fractures in children: intramedullary nailing with immediate motion: a preliminary report. J Pediatr Orthop 1988; 8(4):450–453.

13. Lascombes P, Prevot J, Ligier JN, et al. Elastic stable intramedullary nailing in forearm shaft fractures in children: 85 cases. J Pediatr Orthop 1990; 10(2):167–171.

14. Parsch K. Morote pinning for displaced midshaft forearm fractures in children. Orthop Traumatol 1992; 1:149–158.

15. Yuan PS, Pring ME, Gaynor TP, et al. Compartment syndrome following intramedullary fixation of pediatric forearm fractures. J Pediatr Orthop 2004; 24(4):370–375.

16. Schmittenbecher PP, Fitze G, Godeke J, et al. Delayed healing of forearm shaft fractures in children after intramedullary nailing. J Pediatr Orthop 2008; 28(3):303–306.

17. Lascombes P, Haumont T, Journeau P. [Centromedullary nailing for fracture of both forearm bones in children and adolescents]. Rev Chir Orthop Reparatrice Appar Mot 2006; 92(6):615–622.

18. Rang M. The story of orthopaedics. Philadelphia: WB Saunders; 2000:407–408.

19. Bado JL. The Monteggia lesion. Clin Orthop Relat Res 1967; 50:71–86.

20. Stanley E, de la Garzia J. Monteggia fracture dislocation in children. In: Beaty JH, Kasser JR, eds. Rockwood & Wilkins: Fractures in Children, 5th ed. Philadelphia: Lippincott Williams & Wilkins; 2002:529–562.

21. Wiley JJ, Galey JP. Monteggia injuries in children. J Bone Joint Surg Br 1985; 67(5):728–731.

22. Olney BW, Menelaus MB. Monteggia and equivalent lesions in childhood. J Pediatr Orthop 1989; 9(2):219–223.

23. Letts M, Locht R, Wiens J. Monteggia fracture dislocations in children. J Bone Joint Surg Br 1985; 67 :724–727.

24. Tompkins DG. The anterior Monteggia fracture: observations on etiology and treatment. J Bone Joint Surg Am 1971; 53(6):1109–1114.

25. Kalamchi A. Monteggia fracture-dislocation in children. Late treatment in two cases. J Bone Joint Surg 1986; 68(4):615–619.

26. Storen G. Traumatic dislocation of radial head as an isolated lesion in children. Acta Orthop Scand 1959; 116:144–147.

27. Miles KA, Finlay DB. Disruption of the radiocapitellar line in the normal elbow. Injury 1989; 20(6):365–367.

28. Dormans JP, Rang M. The problem of Monteggia fracture-dislocations in children. Orthop Clin of North Am 1990; 21(2):251–256.

29. Fowles JV, Sliman N, Kassab MT. The Monteggia lesion in children. Fracture of the ulna and dislocation of the radial head. J Bone Joint Surg 1983; 65(9):1276–1282.

30. Ring D, Waters PM. Operative fixation of Monteggia fractures in children. J Bone Joint Surg Br 1996; 78(5):734–739.

31. Ring D, Jupiter JB, Waters PM. Monteggia fractures in children and adults. J Am Acad Orthop Surg 1998; 6(4):215–224.

32. Haddad FS, Manktelow AR, Sarkar JS. The posterior Monteggia: a pathological lesion? Injury 1996; 27(2):101–102.

33. Lloyd-Roberts G, Bucknill T. Anterior dislocation of the radial head in children: aetiology, natural history and management. J Bone Joint Surg Br 1977; 59(4):402–407.

34. Best TN. Management of old unreduced Monteggia fracture dislocations of the elbow in children. J Pediatr Orthop 1994; 14(2):193–199.

35. Bell Tawse AJ. The treatment of malunited anterior Monteggia fractures in children. J Bone Joint Surg Br 1965; 47(4):718–723.

36. Bouyala JM, Christian P, Ramaherison P. [High osteotomy of the ulna in the treatment of residual anterior dislocation following Monteggia fracture (author's trans)]. Chir Pediatr 1978; 19(3):201–203.

37. Stoll TM, Willis RB, Paterson DC. Treatment of the missed Monteggia fracture in the child. J Bone Joint Surg Br 1992; 74(3):436–440.

38. Inoue G, Shionoya K. Corrective ulnar osteotomy for malunited anterior Monteggia lesions in children. 12 patients followed for 1–12 years. Acta Orthop Scand 1998; 69(1):73–76.

39. Lädermann A, Ceroni D, Lefèvre Y, et al. Surgical treatment of missed Monteggia lesions in children. J Child Orthop 2007; 1:237–242.

40. Exner GU. Missed chronic anterior Monteggia lesion. Closed reduction by gradual lengthening and angulation of the ulna. J Bone Joint Surg Br 2001; 83(4):547–550.

41. Hasler CC, von Laer L, Hell AK. Open reduction, ulnar osteotomy and external fixation for chronic anterior dislocation of the head of the radius. J. Bone Joint Surg Br 2005; 87:88–94.

42. Rodgers WB, Waters PM, Hall JE. Chronic Monteggia lesions in children. Complications and results of reconstruction. J Bone Joint Surg 1996; 78(9):1322–1329.

Chapter 8

Wrist and Hand Fractures

Malcolm F. Macnicol and Klaus Parsch

Children sustain fractures of the wrist and hand because they are vulnerable parts of the body during everyday activity, particularly in the older child. Distal forearm fractures account for 40% while phalangeal fractures account for 20% of all paediatric fractures [1]. Twenty-five percent of phalangeal fractures are physeal [2], second only to the distal forearm and wrist. Emergency staff will therefore find themselves dealing with these fractures on a regular basis, ideally with both efficient and knowledgeable help from orthopaedic and plastic surgical colleagues.

Distal Radial Fractures

These fractures dominate paediatric skeletal injury and may be associated with more proximal upper limb fractures, such as the supracondylar humeral [3], or with a scaphoid fracture. The distal ulna often fractures concomitantly, whether at the distal metaphysis, growth plate, or ulnar styloid. It is likely that many of the more minor distal fractures are passed off as a sprain and the child is never referred to hospital.

The different distal radial fractures are as follows:

The buckle or torus fracture resulting from axial compression through the dorsal cortex of the radius. By definition, these are little displaced and stable so treatment is symptomatic with a short arm cast or volar splint for 2–3 weeks.

A greenstick fracture describes a dorsal tilt (volar angulation) of the distal radial fragment, the dorsal cortex bending but remaining intact. In children under 10 years of age angulation of up to 30° can be accepted [4], as this will remodel substantially. However, this decision should be fully explained to the parents and may be unacceptable if the wrist looks obviously deformed.

M.F. Macnicol (✉)
University of Edinburgh, Edinburgh, UK; Royal Hospital for Sick Children, Edinburgh, UK; Edinburgh and Murrayfield Hospital, Edinburgh, UK; Royal Infirmary, Edinburgh, UK

No more than 10° of angulation is acceptable in a girl of 12–13 years or a boy of 14 years. If reduction is undertaken, under anesthesia, a long arm cast is applied with the elbow flexed to 90°. Careful, three-point molding of the cast in minimal palmar flexion and ulnar abduction should be ensured at the wrist and the plaster retained for 3 weeks. This is followed with a short arm cast for 2 weeks [5]. In a randomized study a comparison of short and long arm plaster casts showed equal effectiveness [6]. Radiographic monitoring of the fracture position is ensured for the first and second weeks.

Rupturing of the intact dorsal cortex and periosteum is unnecessary provided padding is minimized and the cast well molded. Forearm pronation is indicated if the fracture presents with volar angulation before reduction, supination for the dorsally angulated fracture.

The complete or "off-ended" fracture is difficult to reduce and 20% displace or angulate in the cast. Reduction relies on increasing the deformity (usually volar angulation) with the distal radius tilted 90° dorsally to allow the proximal and distal fragments to hinge at the fracture site dorsally. A so-called Bier's block (regional intravenous scandicain with tourniquet applied), regional, or general anesthesia is essential for adequate relaxation. Once the cortices are in precise contact the distal fragment is reduced by palmar flexing it, correcting any radial deviation by ulnar tilting.

If contact between the two fragments is anatomical and the reduction feels stable, a molded cast in palmar flexion and ulnar tilt is applied for 4 weeks in younger children, and for 6 weeks in adolescents. Well-molded sugar tong splints are an alternative [7]. The reduction is reviewed radiographically in routine fashion. If there is any doubt about stability following reduction, particularly in the older patient, or if any of the factors detailed below are relevant, retrograde K-wire fixation percutaneously through the radial styloid will secure reduction [5].

Indications for K-wire fixation are as follows:

- bilateral fractures or multilevel upper limb fractures
- open fractures, possibly complicated by neurovascular deficit

- compartment syndrome where a cast will interfere with review
- soft tissue obstruction and unstable reduction
- redisplacement after closed reduction (Fig. 8.1)

Distal Radial Epiphyseal Fractures

The most common is the Salter-Harris type 2, peaking at 12 years of age. The distal ulna is often fractured too. As with metaphyseal fractures, a "dinner fork deformity" is produced, similar to the *Colles fracture* in the adult; less commonly the tilt is volar, akin to the *Smith's fracture*. Small fracture lines may propagate into the metaphysis from the growth plate but are of no significance.

Reduction is usually stable if undertaken early and therefore internal fixation is unnecessary. A well-molded cast in mild palmar flexion is used for 4 weeks. Remodeling is rapid and effective, so residual angulation of 10° is of no concern unless the patient is a year or two from skeletal maturation. As with all wrist fractures the alignment of the radius must be monitored radiographically (Fig. 8.2). Late manipulation of recurrent angulation and displacement is seldom effective after 10–14 days and may be injurious. Salter-Harris types 3 and 4 physeal fractures are rare and may require K-wire fixation after reduction.

Neurovascular complications, largely median nerve compression and compartment syndrome, require acute and effective management. Early recognition and decompression are the responsibilities of the orthopaedic staff. Anatomical reduction and fixation of the fragments are important in preventing this complication.

Premature growth plate closure is unusual, 7–10% according to Lee et al. [8], and possibly iatrogenic if manipulation is forced or delayed. Excision of a bone tether (see Chapter 4), distal ulnar epiphysiodesis, or ulnar shortening

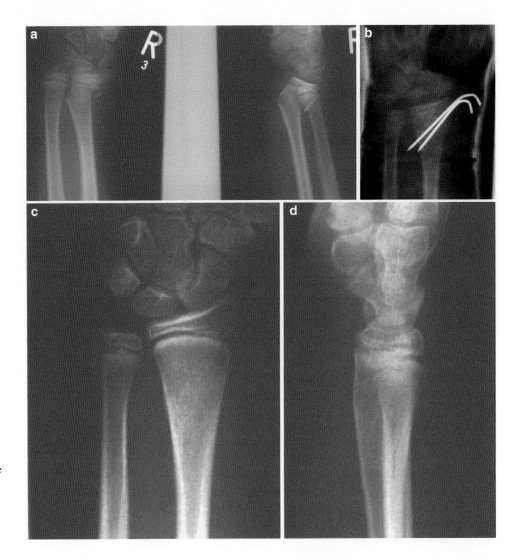

Fig. 8.1 Nine-year-old girl. (**a**) AP and lateral view of distal radial (off-ended) metaphyseal fracture. (**b**) AP view of fracture after closed reduction and stabilization with two K-wires. (**c**) AP and (**d**) lateral views at follow-up after 1 year with normal function of wrist

Fig. 8.2 Thirteen-year-old boy. (**a**) AP radiograph of distal Salter-Harris type 2 fracture of radius and fracture of distal shaft of the ulna. (**b**) Lateral view shows extension fracture dislocation. (**c**) AP radiograph after reduction in cast. (**d**) Lateral view of reduced physeal fracture in a long arm cast, molded with three-point pressure and some palmar flexion. (**e**) AP view of the distal forearm 1 year after the fracture and lateral view of the distal forearm at follow-up

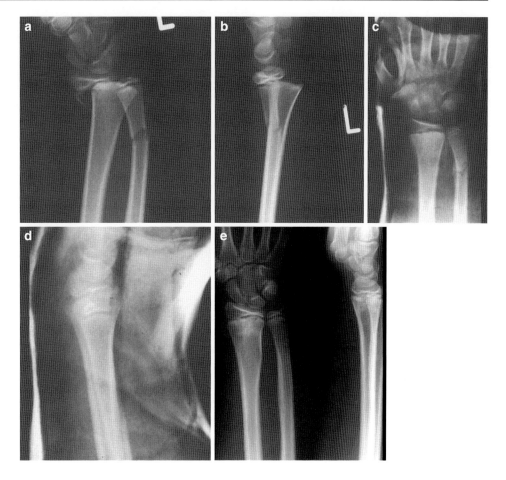

with plate fixation should aim to normalize distal radio-ulnar relationships, function, and range of movement. For late deformity radial osteotomy and possibly radial lengthening may improve function although symptomatic and cosmetic improvement is not assured. Carpoulnar impingement and triangular fibrocartilage tears can be defined by magnetic resonance (MR) scanning. Repair or debridement of the fibrocartilaginous disc may benefit long-term function.

Radial physeal stress fractures (see Fig. 1.18) may develop in gymnasts or from other repetitive upper limb activity. The affected wrist aches and is diffusely tender after exertion, later becoming swollen. Radiographs reveal physeal widening and reactive bone formation. In extreme cases growth arrest occurs.

Distal Ulnar Physeal Fractures

These can occur in isolation but more commonly accompany a distal radial fracture [9]. The displacement is rarely significant [10] and only requires reduction in the older child. Premature growth arrest produces ulnar deviation of the wrist which should be corrected by ulnar lengthening if severe.

Distal Radio-ulnar Subluxation

Forced supination or pronation of the wrist may cause capsular and ligamentous rupture, leading to palmar or dorsal dislocation of the distal ulna, respectively [11]. Reduction is achieved by pronation for the palmar displacement and supination for the dorsal dislocation, maintaining this position of reduction for 4 weeks in a long arm cast with the elbow in 90° of flexion.

Carpal Bone Fractures

The great majority involve the scaphoid (87%), the other carpal bones being injured by crushing or severe disruptions of the wrist [12]. Hyperdorsiflexion may very rarely fracture the capitate. Hamate and hook of hamate fractures may present in athletic adolescents who play a great deal of golf or racquet sports. Lunate fracture-dislocation and lunatomalacia have been reported very rarely in childhood.

Provided the carpal bones are normally aligned on antero-posterior (AP), lateral, and oblique views of the wrist, a short arm cast for 3–4 weeks is sufficient treatment if there is no gapping at the fracture. The wrist should be splinted in slight dorsiflexion and the thumb partially incorporated in the cast, leaving its interphalangeal joint to flex and extend.

Scaphoid Fractures

These are rarely sustained by the younger child but may coexist with a distal radial fracture [13]. Clinical features include the usual history of a fall on the outstretched hand, wrist pain worsened by gripping, and acute tenderness over the anatomical "snuff box." Four-view radiographs of the wrist should be obtained and, even if they appear normal, a precautionary plaster cast is indicated, as for a wrist sprain.

In case of suspicion radiographs should be repeated 10–14 days later if the initial radiological examination did not detect the fracture; occasionally, comparative views of the opposite wrist are justifiable. Failure to splint the undisplaced scaphoid fracture may lead to non-union. However, non-union is more common when the scaphoid fragments are separated and therefore most likely to be recognized on the initial films.

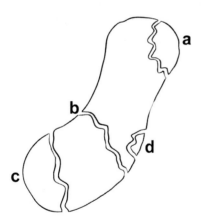

Fig. 8.3 The sites of scaphoid fracture. (**a**) Distal pole, (**b**) waist (*middle third*), (**c**) proximal pole, and (**d**) avulsion

Proximal pole fractures are rare, the majority (75%) involving the distal pole (Fig. 8.3), whether extra-articular or the larger intra-articular fragment, and 25% the waist or middle third of the scaphoid [14]. The incidence rises with age, being negligible under the age of 12 but progressively more common during adolescence. Scaphoid cast support for 4 weeks in the child and 6 weeks in the adolescent almost invariably results in healing (Fig. 8.4). Non-union characterizes late or inadequate splintage in most cases and merits screw fixation via a proximal approach. Additional cancellous bone grafting is essential for the established non-union with separation at the fracture site [15].

Proximal pole avascular necrosis is very rare in childhood [16] and usually progresses to localized osteoarthritis. Regional pain syndrome may complicate the recovery period.

Metacarpal Fractures

Diaphyseal

These are increasingly common as the child matures, usually involving the first, second, and fifth metacarpals. In the shaft the fracture line is transverse, oblique, or spiral and some degree of dorsal angulation and rotation occurs. Angulation of up to 30° is only acceptable at the fifth metacarpal as it is more mobile than the radial metacarpals. Remodeling will eventually correct knuckle recession and prominence of the metacarpal head in the palm.

Mid-shaft angulation of 15–20° leaves functional and cosmetic impairment in the adolescent, unlike the neck fracture, so reduction and transverse K-wire fixation are appropriate.

Reduction is achieved by flexing the metacarpophalangeal (MCP) joint to 90°, then pressing the digit dorsally with counterpressure at the fracture line using regional or general anesthesia. Rotational deformity is unacceptable and must be carefully avoided by reviewing the alignment of the fingers when flexed into the palm. In a few instances open reduction and K-wire or screw fixation are advisable.

Fig. 8.4 Eleven-year-old-boy. (**a**) Scaphoid waist fracture, (**b**) after 4 weeks in a long arm cast with scaphoid immobilization, and (**c**) after 7 weeks the fracture of the scaphoid has united

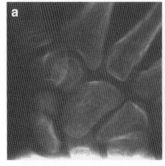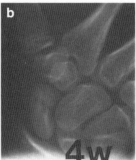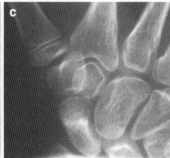

Distal Physeal

These fractures produce dorsal and lateral deviations, usually of the fourth and fifth metacarpals. The type 2 Salter-Harris fracture is the most common; types 3 and 4 carry a poorer prognosis. If the metacarpal head splits, K-wire fixation is advisable.

Reduction is achieved by flexing the MCP joint to 90° and then applying volar pressure to the metacarpal head. This is only applicable to angulations of more than 70° at the fifth or more than 40° at the second and third since remodeling is usually excellent [17, 18]. Avascular necrosis has been reported to result from the intracapsular tamponade [19].

Basal Fractures

These high-energy injuries are accompanied by soft tissue disruption so neurovascular deficit and compartment syndrome should be suspected. If the fracture is extra-articular and involves the thumb, reduction is rarely required. Intra-articular fractures, particularly the Salter-Harris type 3 of the first metacarpal, merit careful reduction and fixation to preserve pain-free motion of the affected joint [20, 21]. The type 2 physeal fracture and minimally displaced fractures involving the other metacarpals can be managed with a 3-week period of volar plaster slab splintage.

Proximal (and Middle) Phalangeal Fractures

These occur when an axial and rotational stress is applied, generally fracturing the proximal phalanges of the index and little fingers. In addition to proximal physeal (types 2, 3, and 4) fractures, the proximal metaphysis, shaft, neck, and distal condyles can be injured (Fig. 8.5). Angulation of the type 2 basal physeal fracture commonly affects the little finger, the so-called extra-octave fracture (coined by the late Mercer Rang, Toronto). Reduction is achieved by a corrective, angulatory force against a fulcrum, such as a pencil in the relevant web space. Although the fracture is relatively stable post-reduction, a volar splint or plaster slab should be applied for 2 weeks, with the MPJ flexed to 70–90° and the interphalangeal joints extended. A further fortnight of buddy taping to the neighboring digit is of value to control malrotation and to initiate movement.

In the adolescent age group avulsion of the ulnar collateral ligament can occur as a skiing injury. Anatomic reduction and fixation by K-wires or a miniscrew are indicated (Fig. 8.6).

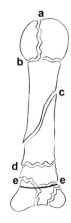

Fig. 8.5 The sites of phalangeal fracture. (**a**) Condylar or head splitting, (**b**) transverse neck, (**c**) spiral, oblique, or transverse shaft, (**d**) proximal shaft, and (**e**) basal condylar or avulsion with growth plate involvement

Shaft fractures are transverse, oblique, or spiral. Any resultant angulation tends to be volar due to the musculotendinous forces. Soft tissue interposition and rotational deformity should be suspected in the more displaced fracture. Reduction should be anatomical followed by the same splintage as detailed above.

Neck fractures are more common than intra-articular condylar fractures. The distal fragment may angulate significantly dorsally [22] so a true lateral radiographic view is essential. K-wire fixation rather than external splintage is appropriate as the post-reduction position is highly unstable and malunion is common [23].

Condylar fractures may involve one or both condyles. Displacement proximally and rotation necessitate accurate reduction of the condyle, often by surgical exposure and internal fixation (Fig. 8.7). Comminution of the fracture poses problems in reduction. Residual malunion leaves angulatory deformity and stiffness of the affected joint.

Distal Phalangeal Fractures

These may be transverse, longitudinal splitting or comminuted tuft fractures, generally produced by a crushing injury and therefore often open. Forced flexion produces mallet finger variants: Salter-Harris types 1, 2, 3, and 4 basal physeal fractures [24] with very occasional extensor tendon avulsion in the adolescent. Forced hyperextension (the "jersey fracture") causes the flexor digitorum profundus tendon to avulse a bone fragment from the volar aspect of the distal phalangeal shaft. Forced hyperflexion may cause a physeal fracture of the distal phalanx, a mallet finger (Fig. 8.8).

A major injury should be suspected when a mallet-type 1 or 2 physeal fracture coexists with a compounding wound. Most commonly encountered in children under the age of 12, a laceration of the nail bed means that the germinal matrix (ungual lamina) is incarcerated at the fracture site. A careful

Fig. 8.6 Twelve-year-old girl.
(**a**) Ulnar collateral ligament
avulsion from the base of the
proximal phalanx of the thumb.
(**b**) The fragment was openly
reduced and fixed by two 0.8-mm
K-wires

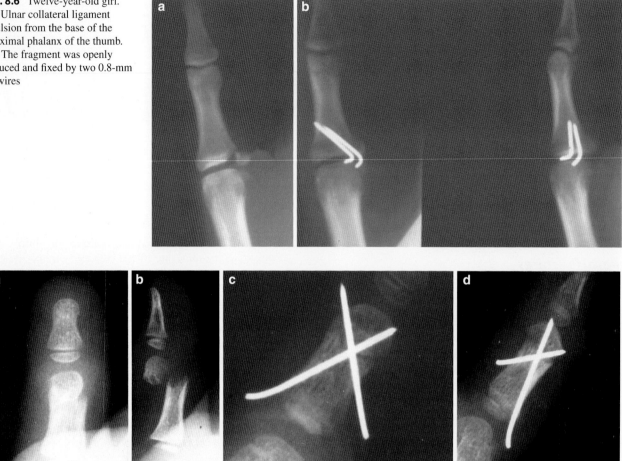

Fig. 8.7 Three-year-old boy. (**a**) AP view of displaced, open phalangeal shaft fracture, (**b**) lateral view confirming complete displacement, (**c**) AP view after reduction and crossed K-wire fixation, and (**d**) lateral view after reduction and crossed K-wire fixation

Fig. 8.8 Twelve-year-old-boy.
(**a**) Lateral view of mallet-type
physeal fracture of the base of the
proximal phalanx of the middle
finger. (**b**) The radiographic
appearance of the injury after
reduction, temporary K-wire
fixation, and union of the fracture

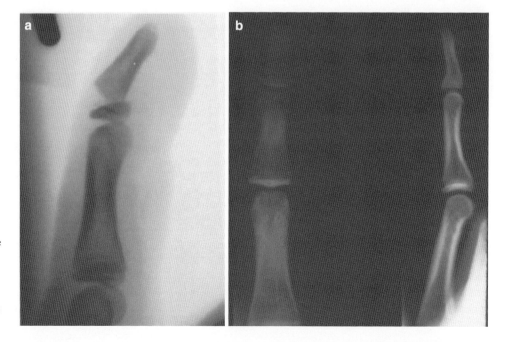

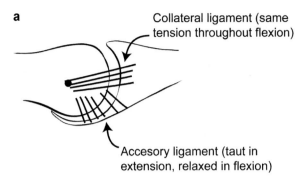

a Collateral ligament (same tension throughout flexion)

Accesory ligament (taut in extension, relaxed in flexion)

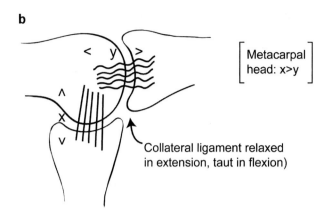

b [Metacarpal head: x>y]

Collateral ligament relaxed in extension, taut in flexion

Fig. 8.9 (**a**) At the interphalangeal joint the collateral ligament maintains the same tension throughout the flexion arc, but the accessory ligament is taut in extension and relaxed in flexion as the volar plate infolds slightly into the joint. Edema will lead to contracture of the accessory ligament if the injured joint is splinted in flexion. (**b**) At the MCP joint the collateral ligament is taut in flexion owing to the cam shape of the metacarpal head ($x>y$), which is also broader in its volar dimension. As there is no accessory collateral structure of concern, the collateral ligament is taut in flexion but not in extension and therefore may shorten pathologically if the injured joint or hand is splinted or bandaged with the joint extended

extrication and repair of this important soft tissue structure is vital [15]. Equally, a subungual hematoma spreading under more than 50% of the nail suggests the presence of a distal phalangeal fracture, possibly complicated.

Volar splintage is effective for most of these fractures once normal anatomical relationships have been assured. The nail should be preserved as a splint and post-reduction radiographs scrutinized. For the unstable reduction or when a Salter-Harris type 3 or 4 fragment remains out of position, K-wire fixation is merited. Contamination of the compound fracture leads to a risk of infection so internal fixation should be used sparingly. When soft tissue loss is of concern a variety of soft tissue reconstructions have been described but are beyond the scope of this chapter.

Interphalangeal Joint Dislocations

These are rare in childhood and usually occur at the proximal interphalangeal joint, the middle phalanx dislocating dorsally. Closed reduction may be achieved by flexion of the joint under regional or general anesthesia, thumbing the middle phalanx back over the condyles of the proximal phalanx. Traction is ineffectual.

Volar plate interposition may require open reduction. This structure spans the joint from the basal epiphysis distally to the volar metaphysis proximally. Damage to the associated accessory collateral ligaments or post-traumatic edema may lead to flexion contracture, so the interphalangeal joints should be splinted in slight rather than major flexion after injury (Fig. 8.9a). In contrast, the injured MCP joint (Fig. 8.9b) should be held in 60–90° of flexion after fracture or significant soft tissue disruption.

Conclusion

Fractures of the hand and wrist are highly visible and disturbing injuries for the child and family. Although many fractures are relatively trivial, experience is needed in deciding when to reduce angulatory and rotational deformities. Internal fixation should be used sparingly and can be avoided if reduction is timely, accurate, and effectively controlled by carefully applied splints and plasters.

References

1. Landin LA. Epidemiology of children's fractures. J Pediatr Orthop B 1997; 68: 79–83.
2. Mizuta T, Benson WM, Foster BK, et al. Statistical analysis of the incidence of physeal fractures. J Pediatr Orthop 1987; 7:518–23.
3. Biyani A, Gupta SR, Sharma JC. Ipsilateral supracondylar fracture of humerus and forearm bones in children. Injury 1989; 20:203–7.
4. Kasser JR. Forearm fractures. In: MacEwen GD, et al., eds. A Practical Approach to Assessment and Treatment. Baltimore: William and Wilkins; 1993:165–90.
5. McLaughlan GJ, Cowan B, Annan IH, Robb JE. Management of completely displaced metaphyseal fractures of the distal radius in children. A prospective, randomised controlled trial. J Bone Joint Surg [Br] 2002; 84:413–7.
6. Webb GR, Galpin RD, Armstrong DG. Comparison of short and long arm plaster casts for displaced fractures in the distal third of the forearm in children. J Bone Joint Surg [Am] 2006 ; 88:9–17.
7. Denes AE Jr, Goding R, Tamborlane J, et al. Maintenance of reduction of pediatric distal radius fractures with a sugar-tong splint. Am J Orthop. 2007; 36:68–70.
8. Lee BS, Esterhai JL, Das M. Fracture of the distal radial epiphysis. Clin Orthop Relat Res 1984; 185:90–6.
9. Bley L, Seitz WH Jr. Injuries of the distal ulna in children. Hand Clin 1998; 14:231–7.
10. Golz RJ, Grogan DP, Greene TL. Distal ulnar physeal injury. J Pediatr Orthop 1991; 11:318–26.

11. Mansat M, Mansat C, Martinez C. L'articulation radio-cubitale inferieur. Pathologie traumatique. In: Razemon JP, Fisk GR, eds. Le poignet. Paris: Expansion Scientifique Francaise; 1983:187–95.
12. Nafie SA. Fractures of the carpal bones in children. Injury 1987; 18:117–9.
13. Greene WB, Anderson WJ. Simultaneous fracture of the scaphoid and radius in children. J Pediatr Orthop 1982; 2:191–4.
14. Vahvanen V, Westerlund M. Fractures of the carpal scaphoid in children. A clinical and roentgenological study of 108 cases. Acta Orthop Scand 1980; 51:909–13.
15. Greene MH, Hadied AM, Lamont RL. Scaphoid fractures in children. J Hand Surg (Am) 1984; 9:536–41.
16. Larson B, Light TR, Ogden JA. Fracture and ischemic necrosis of the immature scaphoid. J Hand Surg (Am) 1987; 12:122–7.
17. Ford DJ, Ali MS, Steel WM. Fractures of the fifth metacarpal neck: is reduction or immobilisation necessary? Hand Clin 1989; 14:165–7.
18. Sanders RA, Frederick HA. Metacarpal and phalangeal osteotomy with miniplate fixation. Orthop Rev 1991; 20:449–56.
19. Prosser AJ, Irvine GB. Epiphyseal fracture of the metacarpal head. Injury 1988; 19:34–47.
20. Kjaer-Peteresen K, Junk AC, Petersen LK. Intra-articular fractures at the base of the first metacarpal. J Hand Surg (Br) 1992; 17: 144–7.
21. Dartee DA, Brink PR, Von-Houte HP. Iselin's operative technique for thumb proximal metacarpal fractures. Injury 1992; 23:370–2.
22. Dixon GL, Moon NF. Rotational supracondylar fractures of the proximal phalanx in children. Clin Orthop Relat Res 1972; 83:151–6.
23. Vandenberk P, De Smet L, Fabry G. Finger fractures in children treated with absorbable pins. J Pediatr Orthop [part B] 1996; 5: 27–30.
24. Seymour N. Juxtaepiphyseal fractures of the terminal phalanx of the finger. J Bone Joint Surg [Br] 1966; 48:347–9.

Chapter 9

Fractures of the Pelvis

Peter W. Engelhardt

Frequency and Mechanism of Injury

Pelvic fractures are uncommon in children [1]. They account for only 1–2% of fractures seen by paediatric orthopaedic surgeons [2]. Their rarity is due to the greater volume of cartilage which provides a buffer for energy absorption. Case reports of pelvic fractures in early childhood are infrequent. Usually fractures of the pelvis are seen in polytraumatized children who have been struck by a motor vehicle. High-energy trauma is often life-threatening because of associated soft-tissue injuries and massive hemorrhage. These take priority over the fracture.

Uncomplicated fractures include all kinds of avulsions of the apophyses of the pelvis. These avulsions occur in children and adolescents playing soccer or football and result from sudden contraction of the muscle which inserts into the apophysis. Fractures of the acetabulum are even more rare and account for 5% of the pelvic fractures in children [3].

Classification

The classification of Torode and Zieg [4] is simple and follows a logical progression of injury status from mild to severe (Fig. 9.1). For practical purposes, fractures of the acetabulum need special attention due to potential injury of the growth cartilage, leading to incongruency of the hip and subsequent subluxation [5].

Type I

Avulsion of parts of the anterior iliac apophysis, the ischial tuberosity (Fig. 9.2) or the anterior inferior iliac spine (Fig. 9.3) represents a chondro-osseous injury, especially in the adolescent athlete.

Type II

Iliac wing fractures occur as a result of direct force against the pelvis.

Type III

Simple pelvic ring fracture, usually involving the pubic rami or disruption of the pubic symphysis.

Type IV

Instability of the pelvis is the result of a fracture or joint disruption creating abnormal motion when stressed or loaded. Included here are bilateral pubic rami fractures, fractures involving either the right or the left pubic ramus or the symphysis, and additional fracture-dislocation of the posterior elements of the pelvis (Fig. 9.4).

Assessment

Fractures of the pelvis need a multidisciplinary approach. Additional injuries of the genitourinary system, the abdomen, and the central nervous system must be ruled out

P.W. Engelhardt (✉)
Department of Orthopedic Surgery, Hirslanden Clinic Aarau, Aarau, Switzerland

Fig. 9.1 Torode and Zieg's classification of pelvic fractures in children. See text for details

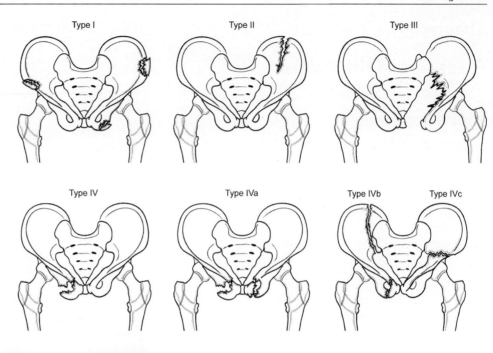

and properly treated. A computed tomography (CT) scan is indicated when there is suspicion of posterior element disruption particularly around the sacro-iliac joint (Type IV). Possible hemorrhage merits consultation with a vascular surgeon.

Treatment

It is generally accepted that children have greater potential for healing and remodeling skeletal injuries. Conservative treatment of fractures of the pelvis is the rule with protected weight bearing and a gradual return to activity [1–4]. External fixation is necessary for pelvic ring displacement of more than 2 cm [2] (Fig. 9.5).

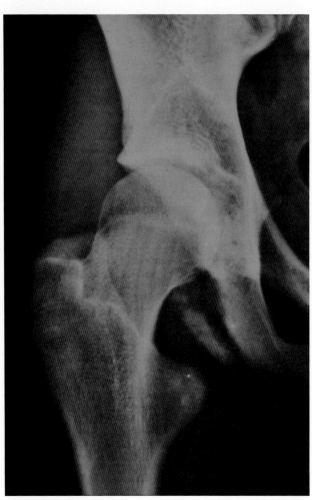

Fig. 9.2 Avulsion of the ischial tuberosity in a 16-year-old skier

Avulsion Fractures of the Ischial Tuberosity (Type I)

Sudden tension in the hamstrings during a fall, for example, in skiing accidents, can cause avulsion of the ischial tuberosity (Fig. 9.2). Initial bed rest is followed by crutch-supported walking. Abundant callus formation can form a pseudotumor, causing diagnostic concerns. Excessive callus formation can be painful and may require excision. Widely dislocated avulsions of the ischial tuberosity should be fixed by a lag screw [6].

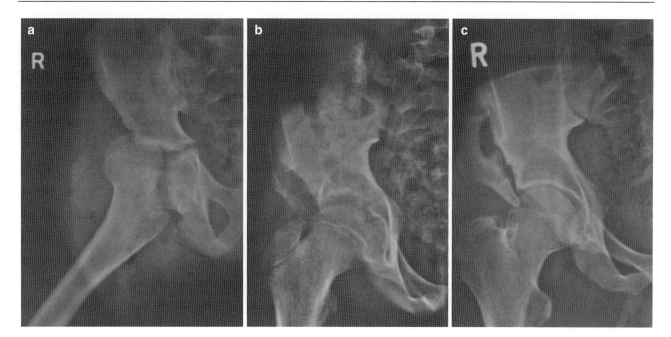

Fig. 9.3 (**a**) Anterior hip dislocation in a 12-year-old boy. The avulsed anterior inferior iliac spine is not visible on the plain film taken immediately after the injury because it is still cartilaginous. (**b**) Ossification of the displaced anterior component of the pelvis after 3 months. (**c**) After cessation of growth a large, ossified fragment persists in the groin, causing symptoms

Avulsion Fractures of the Anterior Superior and Anterior Inferior Iliac Spines (Type I)

Typically, these are sports injuries, for example, when playing soccer or hurdling. The fragment is larger than estimated on the radiograph because of the additional chondal component (Fig. 9.3). In cases with minimal displacement, bed rest with the hip flexed is sufficient. Near the end of growth a severely displaced apophysis may be openly reduced and fixed with strong sutures or with a lag screw.

Marginal Fractures of The Pelvic Ring (Type II)

The strength and rigidity of the pelvis is not affected. Cracks in the iliac wing heal without sequelae. Bed rest until the pain subsides is sufficient.

Anterior and Posterior Fractures of the Pelvic Ring, Malgaigne Fractures (Type III/IV)

Rotational and vertical instability should be analyzed by radiograph or under image intensification. Anterior disruption of the ring heals conservatively. Additional posterior lesions need to be carefully checked by CT scan.

Occasionally, open reduction and the application of an anterior external fixation frame are indicated (Fig. 9.5a). Intra-abdominal trauma or bladder and urethral disruption (Fig. 9.4b) should always be considered and one must beware of misinterpreting a widened symphysis or sacro-iliac joint since the thicker growth cartilage layer makes the interval proportionally wider than in adults. Disruption through the sacro-iliac joint (Fig. 9.5b) can result in severe growth disturbance of the whole pelvis [7, 8].

Fractures of the Acetabulum

These fractures are best seen on CT scans. The potential hazard of premature closure of the triradiate cartilage (Fig. 9.6) must be kept in mind, but may not be prevented by open reduction. Often there is a delay in recognizing compression of the growth cartilage. In Salter-Harris Type V lesions, premature fusion may occur with progressive subluxation of the hip. Thickening of the medial acetabular wall is also observed (Fig. 9.6b). It is doubtful if the adult approach to fractures of the acetabulum should be applied to children. Secondary reconstructive procedures, such as a shelf operation or Chiari and intertrochanteric osteotomies, may be necessary to contain the femoral head [9]. In a survey of 34 patients, 16 were treated surgically because of incongruence or instability [3]. A common cause of acetabular fracture was dislocation of the femoral head, predominantly in a

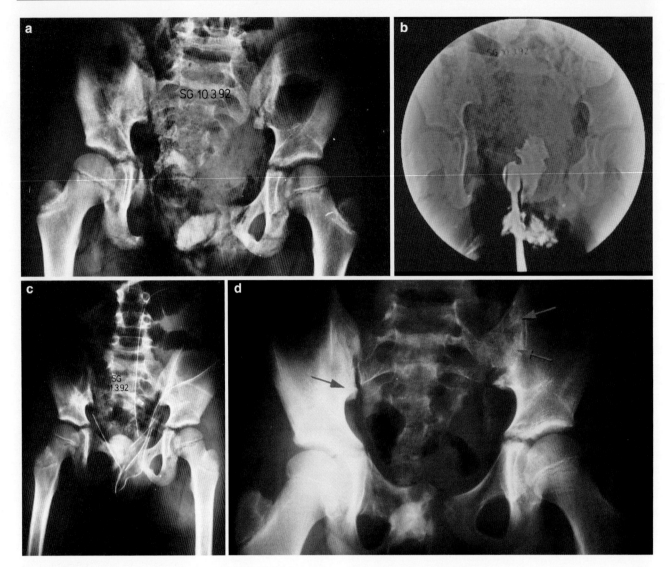

Fig. 9.4 (**a**) A 9-year-old boy was run over by a car causing severe fracture-dislocation of the pelvis with additional intra-abdominal trauma. (**b**) A urethrogram reveals a ruptured urethra. (**c**) Fixation of the pelvic fragments was achieved with heavy-duty sutures via a transabdominal approach. (**d**) Outcome 3 years post-injury. Fusion of the left sacro-iliac joint has not led to problems as yet

posterior direction. The indications for operative treatment were unstable posterior or central fracture dislocations and the presence of intra-articular fragments. Depending upon the fracture type and associated injuries, an anterior or a posterior approach was used.

Outcome

Outcome studies focus mainly on mortality rates with an average of 7.2% due to associated polytrauma. Type I, II, and III fractures usually heal without long-term disability. Initially they need close observation in the presence of additional genitourinary and other soft tissue injury. Disruption of the symphysis pubis heals even in the presence of diastasis because the lesion does not interfere with the growth potential of the cartilage.

Depending on the severity of the skeletal lesion, particularly if combined with vertical instability, permanent disability may result. Injury of the growth cartilage may lead to deformity of the pelvis, with leg length discrepancy and pelvic obliquity as well as fusion of the sacro-iliac joint [9]. In the case of triradiate cartilage damage, a shallow acetabulum can be expected, with the need for secondary reconstructive procedures [5]. Excellent results correlate with the eventual congruence of the reduction. Post-traumatic acetabular dysplasia differs from the morphology of developmental dysplasia of the hip as central acetabular wall thickening is more marked and the acetabulum is retroverted rather than anteverted [5].

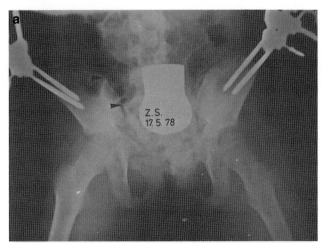

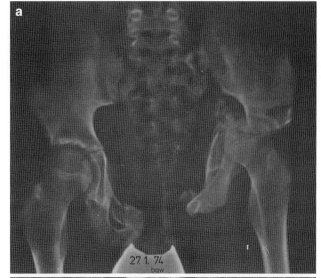

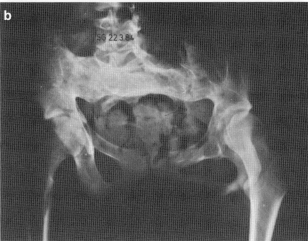

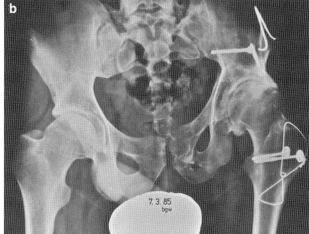

Fig. 9.5 (**a**) External fixator to close the "open book" injury of the pelvis in an 8-year-old child. (**b**) At the age of 15 years, major deformity of the pelvis had developed due to multiple growth plate arrest (including both sacro-iliac joints)

Fig. 9.6 (**a**) High-velocity trauma due to a motorcycle accident in a 15-year-old patient. Major disruption of the left hemipelvis with gross displacement of the fractured acetabulum. Open reduction was undertaken. (**b**) At the age of 27 years, leg length discrepancy and extrusion of the femoral head developed due to injury to the triradiate cartilage. Metal implants have been partially removed

References

1. Widman RF. Fractures of the pelvis. In: Beaty JH, Kasser JR, eds. Rockwood and Wilkins: Fractures in Children, 6th ed. Philadelphia, PA: Lippincott Williams Wilkins; 2006:850–860.
2. Holden CP, Holman J, Herman MJ. Pediatric pelvic fractures. J Am Acad Orthop Surg 2007; 15:172–177.
3. Heeg M, de Ridder V, Tornetta P, et al. Acetabular fractures in children and adolescents. Clin Orthop Rel Res 2000; 376:80–86.
4. Torode I, Zieg D. Pelvic fractures in children. J Pediatr Orthop 1985; 5:76–84.
5. Trousdale RT, Ganz R. Post-traumatic acetabular dysplasia. Clin Orthop Rel Res 1994; 305:124–132.
6. Stiletto RJ, Baacke M, Gotzen L. Comminuted pelvic ring disruption in toddlers: Management of a rare injury. J Trauma 2000; 48:161–166 .
7. Garvin K, McCarthy R, Barnes C, et al. Pediatric pelvic ring fractures. J Pediatr Orthop 1990; 10:577–582.
8. Engelhardt P. Die Malgaigne-Beckenringverletzung im Kindesalter. Orthopaede 1992; 21:422–426.
9. Schwarz N, Posch E, Mayer J, et al. Long term results of unstable pelvic ring fractures in children. Injury 1998; 29:421–433.

Chapter 10

Femoral Neck Fractures

Peter W. Engelhardt

Frequency and Mechanism of Injury

Fractures around the hip joint result from violent force such as high-energy trauma or less frequently in association with pathological conditions [1]. Femoral neck fracture as an atypical presentation of child abuse has also been presented recently [2]. The overall incidence of femoral neck fractures in children is less than 1% [3]. They occur in children of all ages, but the highest incidence is in 11- and 12-year-olds, with 60–75% occurring in boys, about the same age as slipped upper femoral epiphysis (SUFE) has its peak incidence. It is mandatory to identify additional injuries in the polytraumatized child (Fig. 10.1). Age-related differences in the mechanical property of bone account for the greater frequency of hip fractures among adults than among children, the ratio of adult to childhood fracture frequency being 130:1 [4].

A fracture of the femoral neck may be caused by a force applied to the greater trochanter, producing valgus angulation, or from axial loading directed along the shaft of the femur, causing varus deformity. A fracture caused by relatively minor trauma may be indicative of pathological conditions such as a cyst, disuse osteopenia, or neurological disorders. Large series of femoral neck fractures in children have been published [4–6]. Improvements in management and fixation techniques have significantly reduced complication rates over time.

A stress fracture of the femoral neck in a patient with an open physis is rare, so investigations should rule out any underlying disease. The youngest case is reported in a child of 10 years [7].

Classification

Hip fractures in children are classified according to their location and morphology. The AO Classification Supervisory Committee (CSC) coordinated by AO Clinical Investigation and Documentation (AOCID) has set a new standard for the classification of paediatric fractures [8] including proximal epiphyseal fractures (31-E) and the proximal metaphyseal femoral neck fracture (31-M).

The morphology of the fracture (Fig. 10.2) is classified according to the AO method which closely resembles the older system of Colonna and Delbet [9] (Table 10.1).

Assessment

The child is fearful of any passive limb motion and unable to move actively. The diagnosis is confirmed by radiographs, preferably in two planes if this is not too painful. Sonography is useful in doubtful conditions of hip pain in the child. A fracture line or intracapsular hematoma can be detected by ultrasound. With an undisplaced fracture of the femoral neck, the radiograph may not be diagnostic initially. Computed tomography (CT) can be used to assess the degree of displacement and any intracapsular hematoma (Fig. 10.3). A bone scan at 3 months post-injury is also helpful in detecting femoral head necrosis, the most common complication. Magnetic resonance imaging (MRI) detects avascularity earlier (see complications).

Treatment

The principles of management include

- Minimizing potential complications of avascular necrosis (AVN)
- Avoiding injury to the physeal plate

P.W. Engelhardt (✉)
Department of Orthopedic Surgery, Hirslanden Clinic Aarau, Aarau, Switzerland

Fig. 10.1 (a) A 1-year-old polytraumatized boy run over by a tractor. Type I fracture of the femoral neck (epiphysiolysis). Closed reduction was followed by premature closure of the growth plate with subsequent coxa vara. (b) Coxa vara as a result of the fracture (epiphysiolysis)

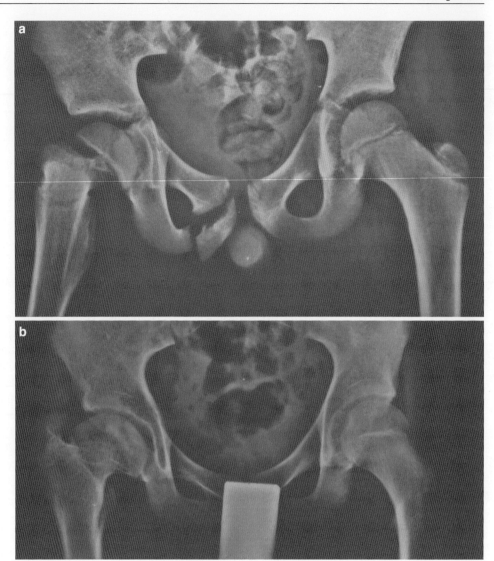

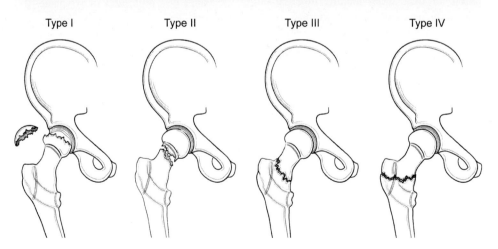

Fig. 10.2 Classification of proximal femoral fractures in the child, according to Colonna and Delbet [9]

Type I   Type II   Type III   Type IV

- Anatomical reduction of the fragments
- Stabilization with pins or screws allowing early protected weight bearing.

Decompression of the hemarthrosis and stable internal fixation are essential aspects of treatment for all fractures with displacement [3, 5, 7, 8]. Undisplaced fractures may

Table 10.1 Classification of Proximal Femoral Fractures

Classification	Location	AO classification	AVN risk	Urgency of treatment	Treatment undisplaced	Treatment displaced	Fixation
Type I	Epiphysiolysis	31-E/1.1–7.1	Very high	Emergency	Eventually conservative	Operative	K-wires, cannulated screws
Type II	Mid-cervical	31-M/2.1	High	Emergency	Eventually conservative	Operative	K-wires, cannulated screws
Type III	Basocervical	31-M/2.1–3.1	High	Emergency	Eventually conservative	Operative	K-wires under 3 years or cannulated screws
Type IV	Transtrochanteric	31-M/2.1–3.2	Low	Delay possible	Conservative	Operative	K-wires or blade plate

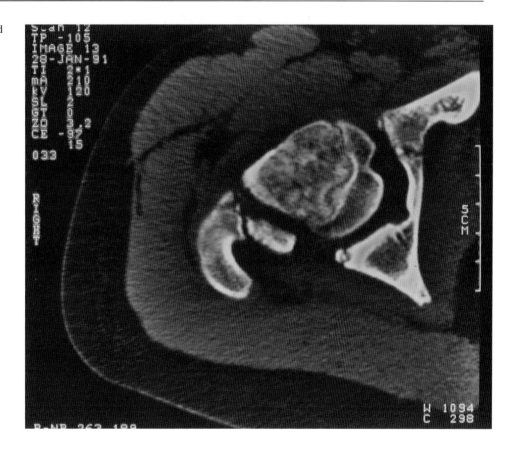

Fig. 10.3 CT Scan for improved analysis of the fracture morphology. Swelling and intracapsular hemarthrosis are mild. Planning of implant size and position is facilitated but a scan is not mandatory

be treated conservatively with cast immobilization using a hip spica. Some authors consider that decompression of the intracapsular hematoma reduces the incidence of AVN [10], particularly the frequency of AVN in displaced fractures [11].

Minimally invasive surgery has a place in undisplaced fractures. Under image intensifier control cannulated screws are inserted over a guide wire in order to maintain reduction. In all other cases the fracture site is exposed using the Watson–Jones' anterolateral approach. An anterior capsulotomy exposes the fragments and their orientation. A K-wire is inserted laterally below the greater trochanter and advanced to the fracture site using an image intensifier in two planes. After carefully checking the accuracy of reduction

the K-wire is driven across the fracture. In type 31-E (epiphyseal) fractures K-wires are inserted into the capital epiphysis and left there while the fracture unites.

In 31-M (metaphyseal) fracture two lag screws are inserted parallel to the K-wire, securing firm and compressive fixation of the fragments without crossing the growth plate (Fig. 10.4a, b). Cannulated screws of appropriate size may also be inserted directly over the guide wires. Shortly before skeletal growth ceases (from the age of 15 onwards) the thread of the screw may be inserted into the capital epiphysis without the risk of major leg length discrepancy from premature growth arrest [12]. The use of several small diameter pins may be sufficient in many cases [6, 13] but can lead

Fig. 10.4 (a) Ten-year-old boy with type III (basocervical) fracture of the femoral neck. (b) At follow-up 1 year after screw fixation solid union of the femoral neck is proven. The epiphyseal plate was not crossed by the thread of the screws

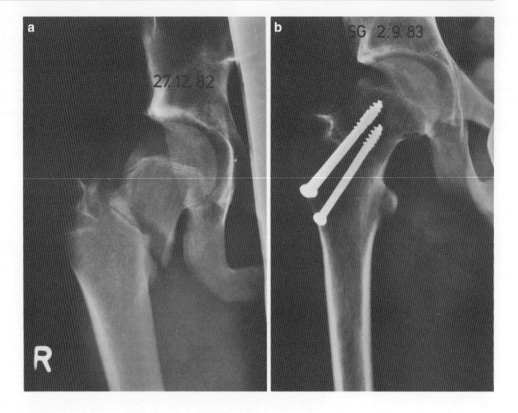

to distraction of the fragments. The large Smith-Petersen nail is no longer recommended for hip fractures in children. It may fail to penetrate the hard bone of the proximal fragment, causing wide separation or comminution at the fracture site. Closure of the joint capsule is not necessary. Immediate post-operative partial weight bearing is possible in the older child. The younger child is kept in bed for 2 weeks and a single hip spica cast can be used to control rotation if there is any concern about stable fixation. Full weight bearing should not be attempted before 8 weeks postoperatively.

Complications

The following complications may arise and determine the late outcome:

- AVN
- Growth arrest
- Coxa vara
- Nonunion
- Osteoarthritis
- Other untoward sequelae.

Avascular Necrosis

AVN, first described in 1927 [14], is the most feared complication because it leads to a very unfavorable result (Fig. 10.5). AVN was seen in as many as 9 of 19 fractures (47%) before the present treatment regimen was established [15]. It is presumed to result from rupture or tamponade of one or both circumflex arteries.

The amount of initial displacement is an important prognostic factor when considering its effect upon the vascular supply of the femoral head and neck but it does not explain AVN after fissure (undisplaced) fracture of the femoral neck. Several authors have suggested that femoral head ischemia results from the hip joint tamponade, which in turn prevents venous drainage [16, 17].

The necrosis can affect the epiphysis alone, the whole proximal fragment, or only the portion of the neck of the femur between the fracture and the growth plate [4]. Epiphyseal ischemia resembles that seen in Perthes' disease [18] and its treatment therefore follows principles that are established for this disease. However, healing and remodeling after post-traumatic AVN in children is usually prolonged and never complete (Fig. 10.5c, d). Decompression and stable internal fixation are the cornerstones of prevention of AVN [19].

Fig. 10.5 (**a**) Transcervical femoral neck fracture with only minimal displacement in an 8-year-old boy. Long-term follow-up after conservative treatment. (**b**) Lateral view of the femoral neck demonstrates the fracture morphology better. (**c**) Thirty months later AVN is clearly evident with collapse of the femoral head which gives a Legg-Calvé-Perthes-like appearance. (**d**) Thirty years after the initial fracture secondary osteoarthritis grade 2 is evident. (Adapted from the archives of the Balgrist Orthopedic University Hospital at Zürich, Switzerland. Used with permission)

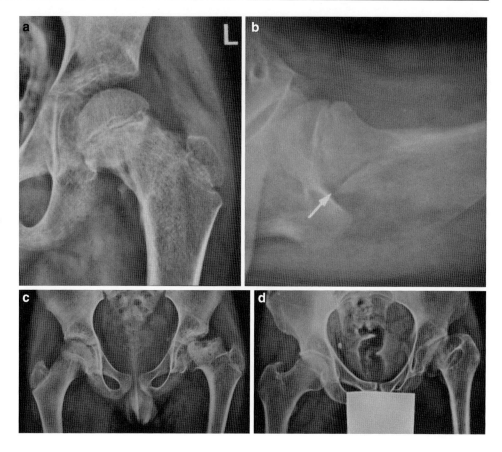

Growth Arrest/Coxa Vara

Coxa vara is caused by premature physeal fusion or by inadequate reduction (Fig. 10.1b). It occurs in about 15% of cases [7].

Nonunion

Delayed healing and nonunion are rarely encountered now that open reduction and stable, compressive internal fixation are recommended.

Osteoarthritis

Secondary osteoarthritis of the hip joint develops as a result of incongruity. Complications in early childhood are usually better compensated for by remodeling than those shortly before skeletal maturity. Deterioration of the hip joint in the form of degenerative joint disease and impaired function may occur insidiously over a period of many years (Fig. 10.5d).

Other Complications

Subtrochanteric fractures at the level of screw insertion are a potential complication if the femoral cortex has been weakened by drilling or after screw removal. Poorly positioned implants may compromise function either as a result of proximal penetration or from prominence of the distal end of the fixation device.

Traumatic Dislocation of the Hip

Traumatic hip dislocation is a rare injury, accounting for 2–5% of all dislocations [20]. Usually, severe violence is required, but sometimes minor trauma can be the cause of dislocation of the immature hip joint up to the age of 10 years [20, 21]. Posterior dislocation is the most common,

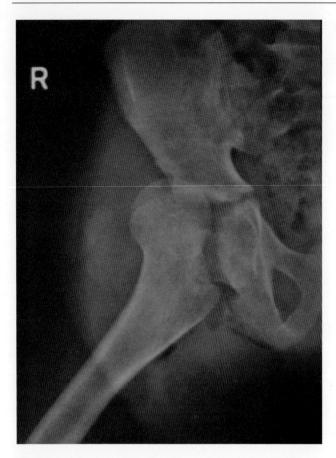

Fig. 10.6 Anterior hip dislocation in a 12-year-old boy (bicycle accident) with avulsion of the chondral physis of the anterior inferior iliac spine (see also Fig. 9.3)

whereas anterior dislocation is rare (Fig. 10.6) [22]. Habitual hip dislocation is reported as a cause of the rare snapping hip syndrome [23] and may occur in Down's syndrome [24, 25].

The leg is held in internal rotation, adduction, and flexion in cases of posterior dislocation. Radiographs should include the whole femur in order to rule out an associated fracture of the ipsilateral femoral shaft.

The dislocation is usually reducible by closed methods. Interposition of small fragments or button-holing of the head through the capsule may necessitate open reduction. Intra-articular fragments are best detected by CT scanning. Post-reduction treatment includes skin traction or even a spica cast if there is concern about stability [20]. The best prognosis results from an immediate closed reduction in the absence of bony or soft tissue interposition. AVN is more likely after violent injury and is less frequent in younger children if the dislocation occurs after minor trauma. Late-diagnosed cases are still encountered in some parts of the world.

References

1. Krieg A, Speth B, Won H, et al. Conservative management of bilateral femoral neck fractures in a child with autosomal dominant osteopetrosis (ADO). Arch Orthop Trauma Surg 2007; 127: 967–970.
2. Gholve P, Arkader A, Gaugler R, et al. Femoral neck Fracture as an atypical presentation of child abuse. Orthopedics 2008; 31: 271–273.
3. Canale ST. Fractures of the hip in children and adolescents. Orthop Clin North Am 1990; 21: 341–352.
4. Ratliff AH. Fractures of the neck of the femur in children. J Bone Joint Surg Br 1962; 44: 528–542.
5. Boitzy A. La fracture du col du femur chez l'enfant et l'adolescent. Paris: Masson; 1971.
6. Canale ST. Fracture of the neck and intertrochanteric region of the femur in children. J Bone Joint Surg Am 1977; 59: 431–433.
7. Ratliff AH. Complications after fractures of the femoral neck in children and their treatment. J Bone Joint Surg Br 1970; 52: 175–181.
8. Slongo T, Audigé L, AO Pediatric Classification Group. AO Pediatric Comprehensive Classification of Long-Bone Fractures (PCCF). Brochure AO Education, Switzerland: AO Publishing; 2007.
9. Colonna PC. Fracture of the neck of the femur in children. Am J Surg 1929; 6: 793–797.
10. Song KS, Kim YS, Sohn SW, Ogden JA. Arthrotomy and open reduction of he displaced fracture of the femoral neck in children. J Pediatr Orthop part B 2001; 10: 205–210.
11. Ng GP, Cole WG. Effect of early hip decompression on the frequency of avascular necrosis in children with fractures of the neck of the femur. Injury 1996; 27: 419–421.
12. Engelhardt P. Epiphyseolysis capitis femoris und die "gesunde" Gegenseite. Z Orthop 1990; 128: 262–265.
13. Miller WE. Fractures of the hip in children from birth to adolescence. Clin Orthop Rel Res 1973; 92: 155–188.
14. Johansson S. Über Epiphysennekrose bei geheilten Collumfrakturen. Zentralblatt Chir 1927; 54: 2214–2222.
15. Davison BL, Weinstein SL. Hip fractures in children: a long term follow-up study. J Pediatr Orthop 1992; 12: 355–358.
16. Kay SP, Hall JE. Fracture of the femoral neck in children and its complications. Clin Orthop Rel Res 1971; 80: 53–71.
17. Soto-Hall R, Johnson LH, Johnson RA. Variations of the intraarticular pressure oft he hip joint in injury and disease. J Bone Joint Surg Am 1964; 46: 509–512.
18. Ogden JA. Skeletal injury in the child, 3rd ed. Berlin: Springer; 2000.
19. Cheng JC, Tangh N. Decompression and stable internal fixation of femoral neck fractures in children can affect the outcome. J Pediatr Orthop 1999; 19: 338–343.
20. Rieger H, Pennig D, Klein W, et al. Traumatic dislocation of the hip in young children. Arch Orthop Trauma Surg 1991; 110: 114–117.
21. Pearson DE, Mann RJ. Traumatic hip dislocation in children. Clin Orthop Rel Res 1973; 92: 189–194.
22. Macnicol MF. The Scottish incidence of traumatic dislocation of the hip in childhood. J Pediatr Orthop [B] 2000; 9: 212–216.
23. Stuart PR, Epstein HP. Habitual hip dislocation. J Pediatr Orthop 1991; 11: 541–542.
24. Aprin H, Zink WP, Hall JE. Management of dislocation of the hip in Down's syndrome. J Pediatr Orthop 1985; 5: 428–431.
25. Greene WB. Closed treatment of hip dislocation in Down's syndrome. J Pediatr Orthop 1998; 18: 643–647.

Chapter 11

Femoral Shaft Fractures

Klaus Parsch

Incidence and Mechanism of Injury

Fractures of the shaft of the femur including the subtrochanteric and the supracondylar regions account for 1.6% of all fractures in children. The boy-to-girl ratio is 2.3:1, a ratio which may change in the future as girls participate in contact sports like soccer. The incidence seems to have a bimodal distribution with one peak in young children and another in young teenagers [1–3]. The annual rate of femoral shaft fractures has been calculated as 19 per 100,000 children [4].

The etiology of femoral fractures is age-dependent. In the infant, the femoral bone is relatively weak and may break under the load condition of normal tumbles. At kindergarten and school age, about half of femoral shaft fractures are caused by low-velocity accidents like falls from a height, from a bicycle, tree, ladder, or after stumbling and falling on the same level with or without a collision. Due to the rising strength of femoral bone, with maturation in later childhood and adolescence, high-velocity trauma is needed to fracture the femur. Motor vehicle–pedestrian accidents were responsible for these fractures in children from 6 to 9 years and motor vehicle accidents in teenagers. Firearm injuries accounted for 15% of femoral fractures in African-American teenagers in Baltimore. Adverse socioeconomic conditions were significantly associated with higher rates of fracture [5].

Fractures of the femoral shaft from *birth trauma* are rare, with the exception of those encountered in *arthrogryposis multiplex congenita*, myelomeningocele, and osteogenesis imperfecta. Rigid contractures of hips and knees in arthrogrypotic children may cause a femoral shaft fracture during delivery or during later handling (see Chapter 7 of Children's Neuromuscular Disorders). The other risk groups are newborns with neuromuscular disease such as myelomeningocele, osteopenia, and *osteogenesis imperfecta* causing multiple fractures (see Chapters 6 and 7 of General Principles of Children's Orthopaedic Disease).

Femoral shaft fractures during the first 12 months of life are rare. As many as 30–50% may be *non-accidental* from child abuse [6]. It is easy to underestimate this cause and initial assessment by a designated doctor in child protection is important [7]. This risk drops considerably after walking age, with only 2.6% in the pre-school age group [8] (see Chapter 5).

Classification

Paediatric femoral shaft fractures are spiral, oblique, or transverse; they can be comminuted or non-comminuted, closed or open. An AO paediatric comprehensive classification of long bone fractures has been developed. The diagnosis includes the distinction between epiphyseal (E), metaphyseal (M), or diaphyseal (D) fractures as well as the identification of child-specific features. The new paediatric comprehensive classification allows exact documentation and comparison of methods of treatment in clinical practice as well as prospective clinical studies (Fig. 11.1). A complete midshaft fracture of the femur has the following codes: 33-D/3.1 bone 3 (femur), segment 3 (midshaft), type D (diaphysis), child code 3 (complete), severity code 1 (simple) [9].

Clinical Findings

The common signs of femoral shaft fracture are pain, shortening, angulation, swelling, and crepitus. A child with a fresh femoral fracture is unable to stand or walk. The whole child must be examined including the lower leg and pelvic ring and the abdomen so as not to overlook tibial, pelvic, abdominal, or kidney trauma.

K. Parsch (✉)
Orthopaedic Department, Pediatric Centre Olgahospital, Stuttgart, Germany

Fig. 11.1 AO comprehensive classification of paediatric long bone fractures [9]: bone 3 (femur), segment 3 (midshaft), type D (diaphysis), child code 3 (complete), severity code 1 (simple). A complete midshaft fracture of the femur has the code: 33-D/3.1

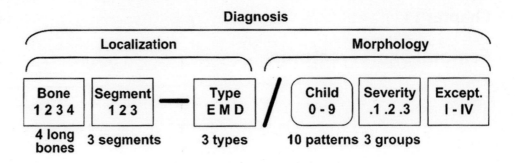

Radiographic Findings

The radiographic examination should include the whole length of the femur in two planes and the adjacent pelvic ring as well as the knee joint. If there is any doubt, the lower leg should be included in the examination. Computed tomography (CT) or magnetic resonance imaging (MRI) scans are not normally needed. The indication for an MRI would be a suspected occult or stress fracture, or a ligament injury of the knee.

Treatment

Femoral shaft fractures are treated according to the child's age and size, concomitant injuries such as head injury or polytrauma, or the presence of open lesions with vessel and nerve injury. Compliance with treatment and socioeconomic factors should be considered.

Femoral Shaft Fracture During the First Year of Life

In the postnatal period a simple cotton bandage or a harness used for dysplastic hips can be applied for a period of 2 weeks.

Bilateral overhead traction has been the treatment of choice for many years. The child has to be in hospital for about 10–14 days. The average transverse fracture heals with a shortening of several millimeters. In a case of suspected non-accidental injury, hospitalization offers the opportunity to investigate the social situation of the child.

Our Preferred Treatment

A *spica cast* after closed reduction of the femoral fracture is the treatment of choice for most paediatric orthopaedic surgeons. The position of the fractured leg is controlled by 90°

of hip and knee flexion [4]. The author prefers a well-padded spica cast with 60° hip and 60° knee flexion. In order to avoid secondary varus deformity, the fractured leg is kept in neutral abduction, while the contralateral side can be in abduction to allow nappy changes to take place. Routine radiographs in two planes after application of the cast are advised. If the mother or the family is well informed about the care of a baby in a spica cast, the child does not need to stay in hospital. During a visit to the clinic after 1 week, routine radiographs will detect angular deviation. Wedging of the cast may be necessary. Due to rapid callus formation consolidation occurs within 2–3 weeks (Fig. 11.2). After removal of the cast restoration of function is rapid.

The *Pavlik harness* used for a period of 3–5 weeks is an alternative treatment for the very small baby. The application does not need general anesthesia and hospitalization time can be minimized. Compliance problems seem to be rare [10].

Vertical traction for femoral fractures in this age group is popular in many places. However, it is less convenient for the child and the family and adds to the cost of hospitalization [11].

Femoral Shaft Fracture from 1 to 4 Years

Traction is still widely used for femoral shaft fractures in pre-school and early for school age children. Hospital stays of 4–6 weeks are usually necessary. Overhead skin traction has the risk of adverse effects on limb circulation [12]. Proximal tibial skeletal traction avoids too much shortening. Pins must be placed horizontally to avoid differences of the intercondylar angle [13, 14]. Traction can be started in the hospital and continued at home but compliance problems and economic considerations are important [15].

Elastic intramedullary nails or intramedullary Kirschner wires are occasionally used for femoral fractures in the pre-school age group. The main indication is failed conventional treatment in a spica cast [16]. Two millimeter-diameter titanium nails are introduced from the medial and lateral metaphysis of the distal femur in order to achieve an intramedullary stabilization of the fracture. The main advantage of this treatment is the opportunity of early mobilization

Fig. 11.2 (**a**) A 6month-old girl with left mid-shaft transverse fracture. (**b**) Child in a 60/60° spica cast with cyclist pants on non-fractured side. (**c**) fractured left femur in the cast. (**d**) Left femur at age 7 months with good callus formation (**e**) Standing X-ray at 18 months. There is minor varus and equal leg-length

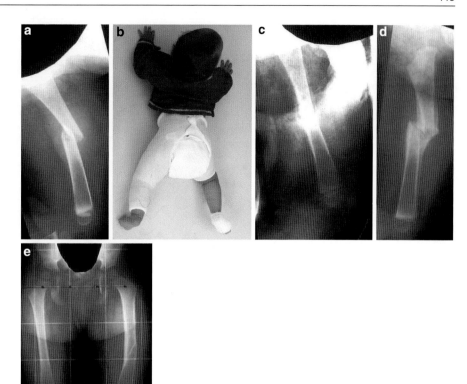

and weight bearing. The consolidation time is short, ranging from 2 to 5 weeks depending on the age of the patient. The implants are removed 3–6 months after introduction. As a sequel to anatomical reduction following the use of intramedullary nails, overgrowth of the involved side of 6–12 mm is common in transverse and oblique fractures.

External fixators are the treatment of choice for open fractures in poly-traumatized patients or for segmental fractures, also in this age group [17]. There is a risk of re-fracture after early removal of the fixator with a lack of callus formation. As in all other fixator use, pin tract infections are common and are treated by local skin care and antibiotics. We do not advise treatment by external fixation for isolated and closed femoral shaft fractures in pre-school children.

Our Preferred Treatment

Spica casts as an immediate treatment have gained wide support as the most efficient and well tolerated in any type of femoral shaft fractures in pre-school children [18, 19]. The cast must be carefully applied. Reduction of a transverse or an oblique fracture should be undertaken under general anesthesia, while spiral fractures can sometimes be reduced only with the help of an analgesic. Care is taken to achieve

good alignment axially and to avoid malrotation. This is controlled by anteroposterior (AP) and lateral radiographs after cast application. Gortex or cotton linings can be used to avoid problems from urine or feces. Shortening of up to 15 mm can be accepted [4]. Generally the cast is worn for 4–6 weeks depending on the type of fracture and the age of the patient. Overgrowth after consolidation will compensate for most or all of the initial shortening (Fig. 11.3).

Femoral Shaft Fractures from 5 to 15 Years

Traction is still widely used mainly in places where there is no economic problem with prolonged hospitalization. Skeletal traction through a distal femoral pin on the fractured side is a low-risk treatment. Traction for 6–8 weeks exclusively and traction for 3–4 weeks followed by a period of 2–3 weeks in a spica cast are the alternatives [4, 20]. Traction with pins through both distal femurs and the child lying on a frame has been popular in Europe during the second part of the last century. Treatment on the *Weber frame* allowed optimal control of rotation, but meant an average period of 4 weeks in the hospital followed by another 2 weeks in a spica before mobilization was started [21].

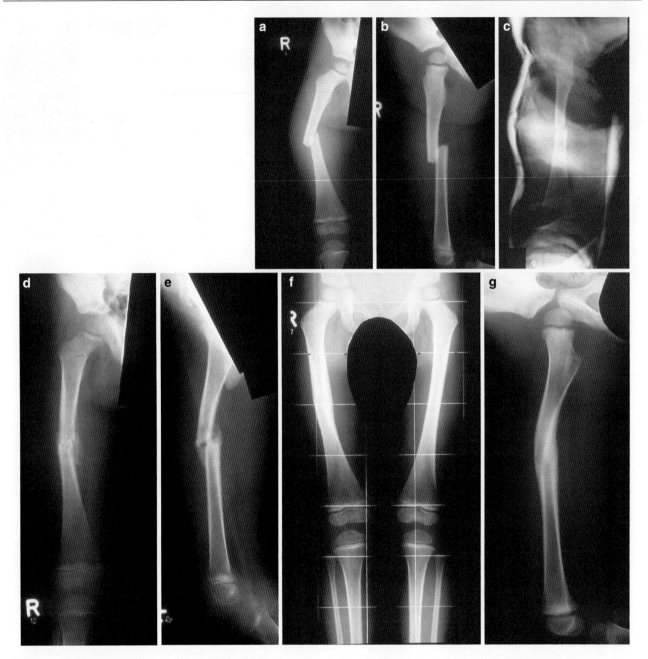

Fig. 11.3 (**a**) and (**b**) Right midshaft transverse fracture of a three-year-old boy. (**c**) AP view of fracture after closed reduction immobilized in a spica cast. (**d**) and (**e**) AP and lateral view of the fracture, slight varus and antecurvatum. sufficient callus formation. (**f**) Standing X-ray of both femora showing residual varus. (**g**) Side view of left femur with good alignment after remodelling of antecurvatum

Immediate spica cast application is a low-risk treatment used in some centers, at least in the age group up to 7 years [22] or up to 10 years [23]. Application of a well-fitting and well-functioning spica cast in a school child is not an easy task. A spica table must be available. Malposition in varus and/or external malrotation must be avoided. Flexion of 45° at the hip and knee joint is sufficient for the older child. The contralateral side needs abduction for toilet care, while the fractured side is positioned in neutral or only minor abduction. Post-reduction the fracture must be radiographed

in two planes. In case of malposition, wedging of the cast may be necessary. Transverse and oblique fractures may develop some shortening [24]. The cast is removed after 6–8 weeks. Most children do not require physical therapy after the removal of the cast and can return to normal activities after 3–4 weeks [25]. There may be compliance problems for some children and parents, especially if they hear about the alternatives of early mobilization with other protocols.

An alternative to cast treatment has been the use of a *cast brace* [26] and a *three-point fixation walking spica* [27]. Both

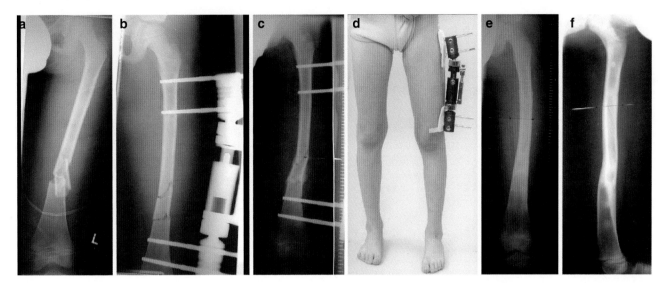

Fig. 11.4 (**a**) Eight-year-old boy with comminuted fracture of left femur and large third fragment. (**b**) After closed reduction of the fracture and fixation with external fixator. (**c**) Left femur after 4 weeks in the fixator. Some callus formation. (**d**) the patient 4 weeks later standing with his Orthofix external fixator. Eight months after trauma and 4 months after the removal of external fixator. (**e**) and (**f**) AP and lateral view of the left femur 8 months after injury. Minimal varus and overgrowth of 7 mm

methods avoid prolonged hospitalization and allow treatment at home.

External fixators of different design (AO, Orthofix, and others) have become popular around the world during the past 15 years (Fig. 11.4). Stable fixation of the fracture allows early weight bearing and return to school [28, 29].

There can be compliance problems in connection with screws and pins. Pin tract infections are less common than when using external fixators for leg lengthening. In transverse fractures the fixator must remain in place for 3 months, while spiral fractures are stable after 2 months or less. Re-fracture after fixator removal may occur in up to 10% of cases causing a second period of morbidity [30–32]. With the advantages seen in the use of intramedullary titanium nails for femoral shaft fractures in children, external fixators have lost ground during the past 10 years, at least for "simple" closed fractures [33].

External fixation still has a place in the extremely rare Gustilo 2 and 3 open fractures of the femur in children, for example, after gun shot or explosion injuries, while Gustilo 1 injuries are better treated with intramedullary nails. [34].

Plate fixation with dynamic compression has been used for many years, especially for polytrauma patients but also in simple closed fractures [17, 35, 36]. With the introduction of intramedullary elastic nails and external fixators, plate fixation of shaft fractures has become less popular and indicated only if other devices are not available.

Submuscular bridge plating as a minimally invasive method has been introduced for complex paediatric shaft fractures but mainly in adolescents [37, 38].

Our Preferred Method

In some centers *elastic intramedullary titanium or stainless steel nails* have become the treatment of choice for standard femoral shaft fractures in school children. The French paediatric orthopaedic schools of Nancy and Metz introduced the so-called elastic stable nails to stabilize femoral shaft fractures, also called "Nancy nails" or ESIN (elastic stable intramedullary nailing) [39–41]. The system spread to Europe [41–45] and North America and is now the treatment of choice around the world [46, 47].

When using elastic nails the child should be placed on a traction table with boots that can be adjusted to the size of the patient's foot. For closed manipulation an image intensifier is necessary. The fracture is reduced by gentle traction and manipulation. In a retrograde manner the two nails are pushed up the medullary canal, the medial nail into the femoral neck, and the lateral nail into the greater trochanter (Fig. 11.5). The retrograde method is satisfactory for all midshaft and proximal shaft fractures, while antegrade insertion is best for distal fractures. The intramedullary system offers axial and rotatory stability [40, 41].

Early mobilization after ESIN fixation of the femoral shaft fracture is possible. After correct implantation of titanium nails assisted walking can start immediately. Full weight bearing is encouraged as soon as the child is able to do so. This varies from 2 to 3 weeks and up to 10 weeks in other centers [48].

Distal femoral shaft fractures are best treated by antegrade titanium elastic stable nails [41]. After reduction of the fracture on the orthopaedic table, two nails are passed distally

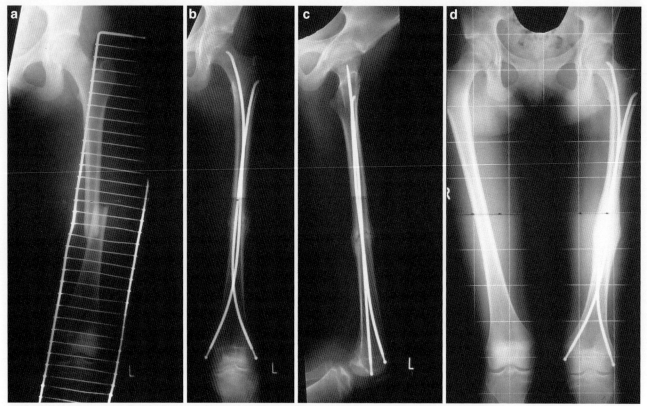

Fig. 11.5 (**a**) Thirteen-year-old girl with left midshaft transverse fracture with shortening. (**b**) Two months after intramedullary titanium pinning. Callus formation on AP view. (**c**) Two months after intramedullary titanium pinning. Callus formation on lateral view. (**d**) Scanogram of the femora at 14 years of age. Full stability from callus before pin removal. The left femur had been shorter before the accident. It is 1 cm short after fracture healing

Fig. 11.6 (**a**) Nine-year-old boy with distal transverse fracture. (**b**) After anterograde pinning with two 3.5 mm titanium nails. AP and lateral views. (**c**) Six months later complete union of the distal femoral fracture, before pin removal

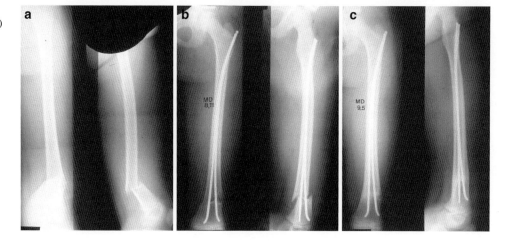

from a subtrochanteric entry point aligning the distal fracture. The distal end of the nails should spread out medially and laterally in order to secure stability inside the marrow space (Fig. 11.6).

Comminuted fractures benefit from additional immobilization in a spica cast, at least in the early phase until some callus has formed. In comminuted fractures, we advise delayed weight bearing in order to avoid secondary malposition and further intervention.

Consolidation is amazingly fast as fracture callus is stimulated by the elastic stability of the nails. The nails are removed after 4–6 months depending on the age of the child. Overgrowth of the fractured femur is common and averages 0.6 cm. The highest rate of overgrowth is seen in midshaft transverse fractures in the younger age group around 7 years. The lowest is encountered in long spiral fractures.

Complications in ESIN treated children are associated with the learning curve of the surgeon [47].

Skin and subcutaneous irritations around the knee, even nail erosions, have been encountered. Problems around the knee account for about half of the complications in titanium elastic nail (TEN) treatment of femoral shaft fractures [49–51]. Skin irritation at the insertion area above the knee can be lessened and even avoided by using a second-generation Nancy nail with olive-like rounded ends (Depuy Orthopedics, Inc.) which will not poke into the subcutaneous tissue, like the cut-off ends of other nails. Olive-ended titanium nails must be inserted with premeasured length [44]. A large assortment of different diameters and lengths must therefore be available. The rounded end is helpful to obtain a hold at the time of removal to obtain a hold on the nail.

Mismatched diameters of the nail, especially the insertion of nails with too thin a diameter, can be the cause of postoperative loss of alignment. The two nails should fill two-thirds of the diameter of the medullary canal. Mismatched diameters may cause secondary malposition and the need for further intervention [50].

Obese children have a higher rate of complications no matter what fixation is used [52]. In a study of 234 femur fractures, children weighing less than 49 kg had a significantly better outcome than those who were overweight [51]. The largest possible nail diameter should be chosen in obese patients [49]. Mobilization, but delayed weight bearing, must be considered in very heavy children.

The use of TENs is widely accepted and has replaced external fixation or plates in most centers. In a prospective randomized study, fractures fixed by flexible nails had a better outcome compared to those treated by external fixation [33]. The complication rate associated with nailing compares favorably with that following traction and application of a spica cast [53].

Flexible steel nails (Ender nails) introduced from below the greater trochanter into the distal metaphysis or by a retrograde approach, from the distal medial and lateral metaphysis into the femoral neck and greater trochanter, have their proponents [54–56].

Intramedullary stable nails with or without an interlocking mechanism have been introduced in the treatment of femoral shaft fractures in adolescents. They can be compared to the Küntscher nails used in the 1950 s and the 1960 s. In addition they offer an antirotatory locking mechanism with screws set in the trochanter and the distal femur [57–60]. Interlocking nails allow early weight bearing. Nail removal is undertaken on an average of 14 months post-injury. A risk of partial or segmental avascular necrosis (AVN) of the femoral head of approximately 10% has been reported. This is caused by injury to the posterior superior ascending branch of the medial circumflex artery [61, 62]. We are in agreement with those who advise that rigid intramedullary rodding should be reserved for skeletally mature patients [63]. They can be used for the very heavy adolescent, where elastic nails may be too weak.

References

1. Landin LA. Fracture patterns in children. Analysis of 8682 fractures with special reference to incidence, etiology and secular changes in Swedish urban population 1950–1979. Acta Orthop Scand Suppl 1983; 202: 1–109.
2. Hedlund R, Lindgren U. The incidence of femoral shaft fractures in children and adolescents. J Pediatr Orthop 1986; 6: 47–50.
3. Cooper C, Dennison EM, Leufkens HG, et al. Epidemiology of childhood fractures in Britain: a study using the general practice research database. Bone Mineral Res 2004; 19: 1976–1981.
4. Kasser JR, Beaty JH. Femoral shaft fractures. In: Beaty JH, Kasser JR, eds. Rockwood and Wilkins' Fractures in Children, 5th ed. Philadelphia: Lippincott-Williams & Wilkins; 2001: 941–980.
5. Hinton RY, Lincoln A, Crockett MM, et al. Fractures of the femoral shaft in children. Incidence, mechanisms, and sociodemographic risk factors. J Bone Joint Surg 1999; 81: 500–509.
6. Taitz J, Moran K, O'Meara M. Long bone fractures in children under 3 years of age: is abuse being missed in Emergency Department presentations? J Paediatr Child Health 2004; 40: 170–174.
7. Banaszkiewicz PA, Scotland TR, Myerscough EJ. Fractures in children younger than age 1 year: importance of collaboration with child protection services. J Pediatr Orthop 2002; 22: 740–744.
8. Schwendt RM, Werth C, Johnson A. Femur shaft fractures in toddlers and young children: rarely from child abuse. J Pediatr Orthop 2000; 20: 475–481.
9. Slongo T, Audigé L, Clavert JM, et al. The AO comprehensive classification of pediatric long-bone fractures: a web-based multicenter agreement study. J Pediatr Orthop 2007; 27: 171–180.
10. Stannard JP, Christensen KP, Wilkins KE. Femur fractures in infants: a new therapeutic approach. J Pediatr Orthop 1995; 15: 461–466.
11. Nork SE, Hoffinger SA. Skeletal traction versus external fixation for pediatric femoral shaft fractures: a comparison of hospital costs and charges. J Orthop Trauma 1998; 12: 563–568.
12. Nicholson JT, Foster RM, Heath RD. Bryant's traction. A provocative cause of circulatory complications. J Am Med Ass 1955; 157: 415–418.
13. Aronson DD, Singer RM, Higgins RF. Skeletal traction for fracture of the femoral shaft in children. J Bone Joint Surg 1987; 69A: 1435–1439.
14. Dwyer AJ, Mam MK, John B, et al. Femoral shaft fractures in children—a comparison of treatment. Int Orthop 2003; 27: 141–144.
15. Newton PO, Mubarak SJ. Financial aspects of femoral shaft fracture treatment in children and adolescents. J Paediatr Orthop 1994; 14(4): 508–512.
16. Simanovsky N, Porat S, Simanovsky N, et al. Close reduction and intramedullary flexible titanium nails fixation of femoral shaft fractures in children under 5 years of age. J Pediatr Orthop Part B 2006; 15: 293–295.
17. Tolo VT. Orthopaedic treatment of fractures of the long bones and pelvis in children who have multiple injuries. J Bone Joint Surg 2000; 82A: 272–280.

18. Czertak DJ, Hennrikus WL. The treatment of pediatric femur fractures with early 90–90 spica casting. J Pediatr Orthop 1999; 19: 229–232.

19. Infante AF, Albert MC, Jennings WB, et al. Immediate hip spica casting for femur fractures in pediatric patients. A review of 175 patients. Clin Orthop Relat Res 2000; 376: 106–112.

20. Sullivan JA, Gregory P, Hemdon WA, et al. Management of femoral shaft fractures in children ages 5 to 13 by traction and spica cast. Orthopedics 1994; 2: 567–571.

21. Weber BG. Fractures of the femoral shaft in childhood. Injury 1969; 1: 65–68.

22. Berne D, Mary P, Damsin JP. Femoral shaft fracture in children: treatment with early spica cast. Rev Chir Orthop Repar Appar Mot 2003; 89: 599–604.

23. Ferguson J, Nicol RO. Early spica treatment of pediatric femoral shaft fractures. J Pediatr Orthop 2000; 20: 189–192.

24. Thompson JD, Buehler KC, Sponseller PD, et al. Shortening in femoral shaft fractures in children treated with spica cast. Clin Orthop Rel Res 1997; 338: 74–78.

25. Hughes BF, Sponseller PD, Thompson JD. Pediatric femur fractures: effects of spica cast treatment on family and community. J Pediatr Orthop 1995; 15: 457–460.

26. Gross RH, Davidson R, Sullivan JA, et al. Cast brace management of the femoral shaft fracture in children and young adults. J Pediatr Orthop 1983; 3: 572–582.

27. Guttmann GG, Simon R. Three-point walking spica cast: an alternative to early or immediate casting of femoral shaft fractures in children. J Pediatr Orthop 1988; 8: 699–703.

28. Aronson J, Tursky EA. External fixation of femur fractures in children. J Pediatr Orthop 1992; 12: 157–163.

29. Davis TJ, Topping RE, Blanco JS. External fixation of pediatric femoral fractures. Clin Orthop Relat Res 1995; 318: 191–198.

30. Hull JB, Bell MJ. Modern trends for external fixation of fractures in children: a critical review. J Pediatr Orthop B 1997; 6: 103–109.

31. Weinberg AM, Hasler CC, Leitner A, et al. External fixation of pediatric femoral shaft fractures. Europ J Trauma 2000; 1: 25–32.

32. Hedin H, Hjorth K, Rehberg L. External fixation of displaced femoral shaft fractures in children: a consecutive study of 98 fractures. J Orthop Trauma 2003; 17: 250–256.

33. Bar-On E, Sagiv S, Porat S. External fixation or flexible intramedullary nailing for femoral shaft fractures ion children. J Bone Joint Surg 1997; 79 B: 975–978.

34 Ramseier LE, Bhaskar AR, Cole WG, et al. Treatment of open femur fracture in children: comparison between external fixator and intramedullary nailing. J Pediatr Orthop 2007; 27: 748–750.

35. Ward WT, Levy J, Kaye A. Compression plating for child and adolescent femur fractures. J Pediatr Orthop 1992; 12: 626–632.

36. Kregor PJ, Song KM, Routt MLC, et al. Plate fixation of femoral shaft fractures in multiply injured children. J Bone Joint Surg 1993; 75 A: 1774–1780.

37. Kanlic EM, Anglen JO, Smith DG, et al. Advantages of submuscular bridge plating for complex pediatric femur fractures. Clin Orthop Relat Res 2004; 426: 244–251.

38. Sink EL, Hedequist D, Morgan SJ, et al. Results and technique of unstable pediatric femoral fractures treated with submuscular bridge plating. J Pediatr Orthop 2006; 26: 177–181.

39. Ligier JN, Metaizeau JP, Prévot J, Lascombe P. Elastic stable intramedullary nailing of femoral shaft fractures in children. J Bone Joint Surg 1988; 70B: 74–77

40. Metaizeau JP. L'ostéosynthèse chez l'enfant. Embrochage centromédullaire élastique stable. Sauramps, Montpellier 1988: 77–84.

41. Lascombe P, Métaizeau JD. Fracture du femur. In: Lascombe P, ed. Embrochage centromédullaire élastique stable. Issy-les-Moulineaux: Elsevier Masson SAS; 2006: 207–240.

42. Dietz HG, Schmittenbecher PP, Illing P. Intramedulläre Osteosynthese am Oberschenkel. In: Intramedulläre Osteosynthese im Wachstumsalter. München: Urban & Schwarzenberg; 1997: 135–168.

43. Mazda K, Khairouni A, Pennecot GF, et al. Closed flexible intramedullary nailing of the femoral shaft fractures in children. J Pediatr Orthop B 1997; 6: 198–202.

44. Parsch K. Modern trends in internal fixation of femoral shaft fractures in children. A critical review. J Pediatr Orthop Part B 1997; 6: 117–125.

45. Till H, Huettl B, Knorr P, et al. Elastic stable intramedullary nailing (ESIN) provides good long-term results in pediatric long bone fractures. Eur J Pediatr Surg 2000; 10: 319–322.

46. Carey TP, Galpin RD. Flexible intramedullary nail fixation of pediatric femoral fractures. Clin Orthop Relat Res 1996; 332: 110–118.

47. Flynn JM, Hresko T, Reynolds RA, et al. Titanium elastic nails for pediatric femur fractures: a multicenter study of early results with analysis of complications. J Pediatr Orthop 2001; 21: 4–8.

48. Ho CA, Skaggs DL, Tang CW, et al. Use of flexible intramedullary nails in pediatric femur fractures. J Pediatr Orthop 2006; 26: 497–504.

49. Luhmann SJ, Schootman M, Schoenecker, et al. Complications of titanium elastic nails for pediatric femoral shaft fractures. J Pediatr Orthop 2003; 23: 443–447

50. Narayanan UG, Hyman JE, Wainwright AM. Complications of elastic stable intramedullary nail fixation of pediatric femoral fractures, and how to avoid them. J Pediatr Orthop 2004; 24: 363–369.

51. Moroz LA, Launay F, Kocher MS, et al. Titanium elastic nailing of fractures of the femur in children. Predictors of complications and poor outcome. J Bone Joint Surg 2006; 88 B: 1361–1365.

52. Leet AI, Pichard CP, Ain MC. Surgical treatment of femoral fractures in obese children: does excessive body weight increase the rate of complications? J Bone Joint Surg 2005; 87A: 2609–2613.

53. Flynn JM, Luedke LM, Ganley TJ, et al. Comparison of titanium elastic nails with traction and a spica cast to treat femoral fractures in children. J Bone Joint Surg 2004; 86A: 770–777.

54. Heinrich SD, Drvaric DM, Darr K, et al. The operative stabilization of pediatric diaphyseal femur fractures with flexible intramedullary nails: a prospective analysis. J Pediatr Orthop 1994; 14: 501–507.

55. Linhart WE, Roposch A. Elastic stable intramedullary nailing for unstable femoral fractures in children: preliminary results of a new method. J Trauma 1999; 47: 372–378.

56. Rathjen KE, Riccio AI, de la Garza D. Stainless steel flexible intramedullary fixation of unstable femoral shaft fractures in children. J Pediatr Orthop 2007; 27: 432–441

57. Beaty JH, Austin SM, Warner WC, et al. Interlocking intramedullary nailing of femoral shaft fractures in adolescents: preliminary results and complications. J Pediatr Orthop 1994; 14: 178–183.

58. Canale ST, Tolo VT. Fractures of the femur in children. J Bone Joint Surg 1995; 77A: 294–315.

59. Gordon JE, Khanna N, Luhmann SJ, et al. Intramedullary nailing of femoral fractures in children through the lateral aspect of the greater trochanter using a modified rigid humeral intramedullary nail: results of a new technique in 15 children. J Orthop Trauma 2004; 18: 416–422.

60. Kanellopoulos AD, Yiannakopoulos CK, Soucacos PN. Closed locked intramedullary nailing of pediatric femoral shaft fractures through the tip of the greater trochanter. J Trauma 2006;60 217–222.

61. Mileski RA, Garvin KL, Crosby LA. Avascular necrosis of the femoral head in an adolescent following intramedullary nailing of the femur. J Bone Joint Surg 1994; 76A; 1706–1708.

62. O'Malley DE, Mazur JM, Cummings RJ. Femoral head necrosis associated with intramedullary nailing in an adolescent. J Pediatr Orthop 1995; 15: 21–23.

63. Letts M, Jarvis J, Lawton L, et al. Complications of rigid intramedullary rodding of femoral shaft fractures in children. J Trauma 2002; 52: 504–516.

Chapter 12

Fractures of the Knee and Tibia

Carol-C. Hasler

Extra-Articular Fractures of the Distal Femur

Incidence and Mechanism of Injury

Distal femoral extra-articular physeal fractures account for 1% of all fractures in children and 5% of physeal injuries. In *hyperextension injuries* the epiphysis is displaced anteriorly while the metaphysis is displaced into the popliteal fossa. The more frequent *varus–valgus fractures* result from abduction or adduction force in the coronal plane. Only a few are Salter–Harris I lesions (Fig. 12.1); the vast majority are Salter–Harris II fractures [1]. In children 2–11 years old these fractures are inevitably caused by severe trauma. In the adolescent, Salter–Harris I and II lesions are caused by less extensive trauma, usually sports injuries [2].

Treatment

In hyperextension injuries the epiphysis is displaced anteriorly; the popliteal surface of the metaphysis is separated only by a thin layer of fat from the popliteal artery. Posterior displacement of the metaphysis carries a greater risk of neurovascular injury. Any severe displacement in the coronal or sagittal plane should be reduced if possible as an emergency bearing in mind the risk of neurovascular injury from the metaphysis in the popliteal fossa [1].

In Salter–Harris type I or II valgus or varus lesions, closed reduction can be attempted by longitudinal traction along the axis of the deformity. Without stable fixation secondary displacement can occur and be the cause of secondary growth disturbance [3]. If there is no substantial metaphyseal fragment, smooth crossed K-wires are used for fixation [4]. If the metaphyseal (Thurston-Holland) fragment is large, one

or two cannulated screws with a washer are inserted transversely to fix the fragment anatomically [5]. If periosteal infolding blocks reduction, open release should be performed followed by screw fixation. The limb should then be immobilized for 6 weeks in a split long leg cast or a splint. The vascular status must be carefully checked both before and after reduction (Fig. 12.2).

Prognosis

If the neurovascular supply is uninjured and compartment syndrome does not develop, the prognosis of distal Salter–Harris I and II fractures is usually good. There is however a high incidence of physeal growth disturbance after distal femoral epiphyseal fractures which may lead to asymmetry of length, angulation, or both (Fig. 12.3). The distal femoral physis has a complex contour which can cause shearing of the fracture line across the physis even in "benign" fractures. If the fracture is sustained toward the end of growth, the risk of post-traumatic angulation or shortening will not be significant. However, if it happens in a younger child the risks of malalignment and shortening are greater. Growth arrest of part or all distal femoral growth plate has been reported in up to 50% of injuries [6–10].

To detect post-traumatic deformity children must be followed closely until maturity [1, 11]. Femoral lengthening with correction of the angular deformity is necessary for children whose deformity becomes unacceptable.

Intra-articular Fractures of the Distal Femur

Fracture Types

Salter–Harris type III, IV and transitional fractures of the distal femur are rare. Salter–Harris type III fractures show a vertical fracture line extending from the physis into the

C.-C. Hasler (✉)
Department of Orthopaedics, University Children's Hospital Basel, Basel, Switzerland

Fig. 12.1 (**a**) Salter–Harris type I fracture of the distal femoral epiphysis of an 11-year-old boy, a pedestrian hit by a motorcycle. The extension fracture was reduced as an emergency. No neurovascular compromise. (**b**) Follow-up at age 13 years. Two years after injury there is premature growth arrest of the right distal femur with 1 ½ cm shortening. Epiphysiodesis of the opposite distal femur equalized leg length discrepancy. Courtesy of Dr. Klaus Parsch, Stuttgart

Fig. 12.2 (**a**) Salter–Harris type II lesion of an 8-year-old girl who had fallen from a tree. (**b**) Lateral view shows posterior displacement of the distal metaphysis. The fracture was reduced as an emergency and fixed with two transverse screws. (**c**) Standing femoral films with the screws still in place. (**d**) Radiological follow-up 4 years later: no sequelae. Courtesy of Dr. Klaus Parsch, Stuttgart

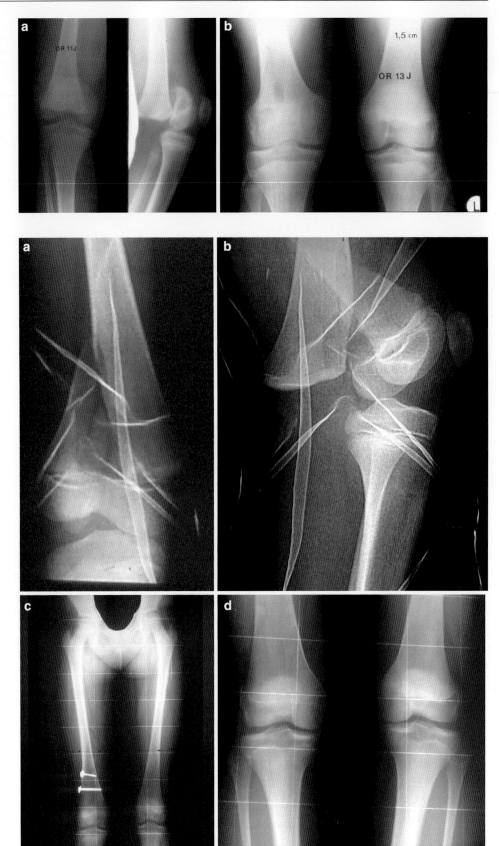

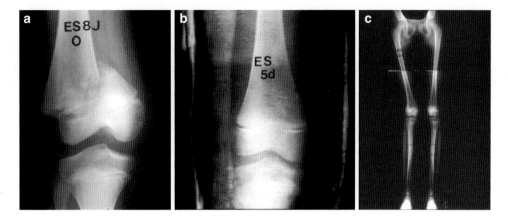

Fig. 12.3 (**a**) Salter–Harris type II fracture of distal femur of an 8-year-old girl run over by a car. (**b**) Following closed reduction in a long leg cast after 5 days. (**c**) Standing radiograph shows shortening and valgus deformity 13 months later. This was treated later by supracondylar varus osteotomy with lengthening. Courtesy of Dr. Klaus Parsch, Stuttgart

joint usually through the intercondylar notch. Type IV fractures run from the metaphyseal cortex, cross the physis, and extend into the joint. As the fracture can reduce spontaneously, it may be overlooked or mistaken for a ligamentous injury. The combination with a physeal injury of the proximal tibia (floating knee) is rare in children. Transitional fractures occur during adolescence when the physis has already partially closed. The asymmetrical closure may allow the non-fused part of the epiphysis to break off with a sagittal epiphyseal and a horizontal physeal fracture line (two-plane fracture) or an additional frontal metaphyseal plane (three-plane fracture). Careful inspection of the lateral radiograph helps to differentiate a transitional fracture from a Salter–Harris type I epiphysiolysis. Correct imaging by radiographs

in two planes and additional oblique planes is mandatory. If available, computed tomography (CT) scans add significantly to understanding the intra- and extra-articular parts of the fracture.

Treatment

Intra-articular displacement is always associated with considerable hemarthrosis and requires anatomical reduction and stable internal fixation with K-wires or screws. Emergency surgical intervention with anatomic reduction may give a satisfactory result (Fig. 12.4), but delayed

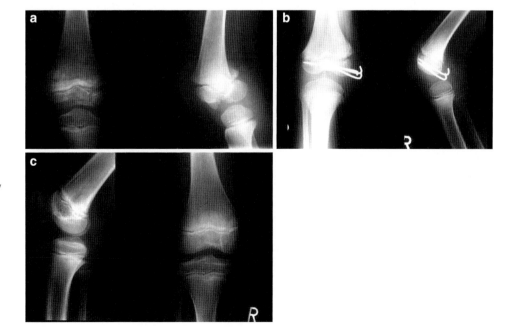

Fig. 12.4 (**a**) Four-year-old boy who had fallen 7 m. Displaced Salter–Harris type IV fracture. (**b**) Open reduction and K-wire fixation of the three fragments. Articular cartilage gap closed anatomically. (**c**) Follow-up 2 years later: full range of motion and intact growth plate. Courtesy of Dr. Klaus Parsch, Stuttgart

treatment has a reduced chance of anatomical reconstruction. Although the risk of an inhibiting growth disturbance is significantly diminished by an anatomical "waterproof" osteosynthesis, partial growth arrest and persistent intra-articular damage may cause secondary incongruence followed by a variable joint stiffness.

The transitional fractures of adolescents should be treated by open reduction and internal fixation. Post-traumatic stiffness caused by incongruence depends on the amount of cartilage damaged by trauma. As these fractures occur toward the end of growth post-traumatic shortening or angulation is less likely [1].

Acute Traumatic Dislocation of the Patella

Epidemiology and Mechanism of Injury

One in 1000 children has a first acute dislocation of the patella per year [12]. It is caused by an indirect external rotation and valgus stress on the flexed knee with the foot fixed on the ground and occurs predominantly during adolescence with a peak at the age of 15 years. Vigorous sports activities, muscular imbalance, relative weakness, and shortening of the thigh muscles as well as proprioceptive deficits during the growth spurt may be responsible. The patient's history allows differentiation of permanent, habitual, or recurrent instability as well as chronic patellofemoral instability from a first episode of true dislocation. In children, patellar dislocation is the commonest cause of acute traumatic hemarthrosis; it accounts for almost half and is also the most likely source of osteo-chondral fragments in the knee joint. Although medial and superior dislocations are described, lateral displacement is by far the most common. Treatment comprises

- immediate reduction of the patella
- recognition and repair of osteo-chondral lesions
- prevention of recurrent dislocation

Clinical Findings

Patients show painful fixed knee flexion and a laterally fully displaced, externally rotated patella. Usually it is easily reducible without anesthesia by gradual passive extension of the knee with the hip flexed to relax the quadriceps muscle. However, most patients present with a spontaneously relocated patella and are unaware of what happened. Some are convinced of medial displacement since the patella-free medial femoral condyle looks prominent. Anterior cruciate ligament (ACL) rupture with subsequent pivoting may give the same impression and needs to be ruled out. Even when the knee cap has spontaneously relocated and the history of trauma is unclear, a thorough clinical examination should reveal the correct diagnosis. Since the medial patello-femoral ligament (MPFL) is invariably damaged by lateral patellar dislocation, local tenderness between the adductor tubercle and the superomedial patella is almost pathognomonic. In addition cartilaginous contusion or fracture at the lateral trochlear border and avulsion fractures at the medial patellar facet may be symptomatic. The hemarthrosis caused by ligamentous and/or osteochondral lesions may be slight or major and develop immediately or slowly over hours.

Radiological Findings

Imaging should include anteroposterior (AP) and lateral radiographs and an axial view (skyline view) of the patella in 30–45° knee flexion if pain allows. Assessment of the patello-femoral spatial relationship is not reliable as long as post-traumatic effusion elevates and lateralizes the patella and delayed imaging is more reliable. Osteochondral lesions may be found at the medial border of the patella as an extra-articular avulsion of the medial rim of the patella (avulsion of the medial patello-femoral ligament), intra-articular at the lateral femoral condyle, and as loose bodies anywhere in the joint. The size of this osteochondral fragment is usually underestimated since only the small osseous part is visible radiologically. The magnetic resonance imaging (MRI) findings are similar to adults and reflect the ligamentous injuries caused by the lateral dislocation and the trochlear damage suffered by the relocating patella: injuries of the medial patellar restraints are found in 81%, simple bone bruises and cartilaginous injuries at the infero-medial patella and at the lateral femoral condyle in 81% and 38%, respectively, and osteochondral fragments of various sizes in 42% [13].

Associated Injuries

The osteochondral lesions are half intra- and half extra-articular. In a prospective study intra-articular fragments were only found after spontaneous relocation when the medial patellar facet hits the lateral femoral condyle on the way back to the sulcus [12] (Fig. 12.5). Arthroscopy is indicated if there are signs of loose *intra*-articular fragments. Some of them are big enough to need open or arthroscopy-controlled fixation. Rarely a large soft tissue gap

Fig. 12.5 Osteochondral shear fracture of lateral trochlear border after recurrent dislocations of the left patella. Finding at open trochleo-plasty for dysplasia

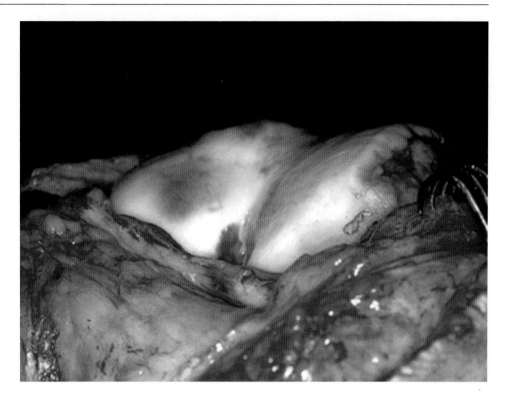

proximo-medial to the patella indicates avulsion of the vastus medialis muscle warranting open fixation.

Predisposing Factors

In most children under 10 years who present after a first patellar dislocation, an underlying abnormality of their static and dynamic soft tissue constraints is found (MPFL, ligamentum patella, patella alta, and dysplasia of the oblique vastus medialis muscle). Bony, ligament, and muscular anatomical factors may predispose to recurrence: Nearly all patients show some radiological signs of patello-femoral dysplasia such as a shallow cartilaginous sulcus, a positive crossing sign on the lateral radiograph or pathologic shape and distribution of the articular cartilage on MRI with consequent false tracking in early flexion [14, 15]. In patients with general ligamentous laxity contralateral patellar hypermobility is typical. It may be associated with hereditary conditions (Down syndrome, Ehlers-Danlos syndrome, osteogenesis imperfecta, Rubinstein–Taybi syndrome, and nail-patella syndrome), poor psychomotor abilities, and contractures of the lateral or central structures of the extensor mechanism. Genu valgum, genu recurvatum, increased femoral anteversion, or increased external torsion of the tibia may also contribute to patellofemoral instability. In most patients there is a unique combination of these factors. Their precise clinical assessment is best evaluated by CT or

MRI, a prerequisite for patients with a first episode of acute dislocation if recurrent dislocation is to be avoided by realignment (See Chapter 8 of Children's Upper and Lower Limb Orthopaedic Disorders).

Treatment

Aspiration quickly relieves the pain of a minor effusion. The fat drop sign in the aspirated fluid as an indicator of an associated osteochondral lesion should not be overestimated. It may also be caused by contusion of Hoffa's fat pad. For the first-time dislocation primary arthroscopy is indicated only if there is radiological or clinical evidence of an osteochondral fragment. After 7–10 days when pain, swelling, and effusion have subsided, a careful examination of the knee joint should be performed to rule out associated injuries of the cruciate ligaments, menisci, and the collateral ligaments.

Immobilization in a cylinder cast or a patella-stabilizing brace for 4 weeks with full weight-bearing will allow healing of the torn medial patellar retinaculum. Early functional rehabilitation with physiotherapy should include range of motion and strengthening exercises, proprioceptive training, and sports-specific exercises for active athletes supplemented by an individual home program. Return to stressful activities including contact sports is allowed when full range of motion and satisfactory quadriceps/vastus medialis (greater than 80% of contralateral side) strength is regained, if there is no longer a knee effusion and no sign of instability.

Operation should be considered for those with osteochondral fractures or persistent laterally subluxated patellae in spite of appropriate rehabilitation [16].

Prognosis

Primary surgical repair or autologous reconstruction of the torn MPFL, medial reefing of retinacular structures, and transposition of the patellar ligament or the oblique vastus medialis muscle do no better than conservative treatment in preventing recurrent dislocation or chronic patello-femoral instability. In a randomized controlled treatment trial in both the conservative and the early surgical realignment groups the rate of recurrent instability was reported to be 46% at 2-year follow-up. By the seventh year, there was a 22% risk of recurrent dislocation and instability episodes were reported as 40 and 45%, respectively [17]. Regression analysis defined the following risk factors for recurrence: young age, female gender, bilaterality, and osteochondral lesions. Recurrent dislocations are therefore most common in immature girls. Half of the re-dislocations occur within 2 years of the first injury [18]. Patients and parents need to be informed accordingly. Chronic post-traumatic anterior knee pain seems to be related to the degree of patello-femoral chondromalacia and warrants further assessment by MRI.

Osteochondral Fractures of the Knee

Mechanism of Injury

Shearing forces on the cartilage may cause osteochondritis dissecans or, if major and acute, a chondral or osteochondral fracture. In acute dislocations of the patella osteochondral fragments may be displaced as the patella strikes the lateral femoral condyle in relocation. Accordingly the lesions are found at the lateral trochlea or at the medial margin of the patella. The latter should be differentiated from an avulsion fracture of the medial patellar retinaculum which is extra-articular. Rarely, a direct fall on the knee or a flexion-rotation injury with major shearing forces involves the weight-bearing surface of the medial or lateral femoral condyle.

Clinical and Radiological Findings

Symptoms may be minimal and a high index of suspicion is required to prevent delayed diagnosis [19]. Clinical findings depend on the severity of the trauma, the size and origin of the fragment, and concomitant menisco-ligamentous injuries. A large osteochondral fragment leads to a significant hemarthrosis, swelling, and pain. If standard AP and skyline radiographs are not conclusive, a tunnel view better depicts the intercondylar area. Radiographs are searched for lesions at the condylar and patellar margins and for free fragments. Small pieces and those with little subchondral bone attached may go unrecognized. The differential diagnosis includes acute osteochondral fractures, impression fractures, chondral flaps, and separations as well as osteochondritis dissecans [20].

Late Presentation

The initial clinical and radiological examination may not reveal a fragment, the fragment is overlooked, or patients present much later. A history of intermittent pain on weight-bearing, mainly during sports, swelling, and transitory locking of the knee should raise suspicion of a meniscal problem or a loose body after an osteochondral fracture, the latter being more frequent during growth. Large, floating fragments are often palpable at different sites, even by the patient, and are visible on radiograph. If the diagnosis is not clear and the radiograph negative, MRI with intra-articular contrast medium (Gadolinium) helps to define the size, depth, origin, and stability of any fragment.

Treatment

Arthroscopic examination and clinical assessment of ligament stability under anesthesia give precise information about the size and origin of the fragment as well as additional injuries. Undisplaced lesions will heal with conservative treatment or, in very active young people, with temporary immobilization. In the fresh injury, fixation should be considered for vital fragments over 1 cm which consist of enough bone and arise from a weight-bearing area. Stable fixation with the implant buried beneath the cartilage can be performed with a Herbert screw, an AO mini-fragment screw, or biodegradable pins or screws inserted either arthroscopically or through a lateral or medial mini-arthrotomy [21]. Smaller fragments (under 1 cm) are removed. After several weeks or months osteochondral fragments lose their original size and shape which renders fixation difficult. Of course removal of the fragment prevents further locking and effusion of the knee. However, if there is a large crater in a weight-bearing area, a procedure to reconstruct the cartilaginous surface should be considered (e.g., osteochondral grafts and microfracturing). The value of those procedures during growth is unclear at the moment and it should be remembered that even large defects may undergo chondral regeneration with satisfactory results in children and adolescents [19].

Fractures of the Patella

Mechanism of Injury

The high proportion of shock-absorbing cartilage explains why fractures of the patella are rare in children. They either occur from a direct blow, mostly a fall on the bent knee, or a forceful contraction of the quadriceps muscle (avulsion fractures and sleeve fractures) followed by pain, swelling, and the inability to straight leg raise.

Fracture Types

The most frequent type is an osteochondral avulsion fracture of the medial border after a patella dislocation. Longitudinal fractures are usually undisplaced and in most cases only visible on an axial view. Transverse fractures and sleeve fractures (sleeve of articular cartilage, periosteum, and various amounts of bone pulled off) at the inferior or rarely at the superior pole show varying amounts of displacement due to the tension of the extensor muscles (Fig. 12.6). They correspond to a patellar tendon disruption in adults.

Sleeve fractures account for half (excluding patella dislocations) of all patella fractures and are therefore the most common during growth. This almost adolescence-specific event should be regarded as an avulsion injury and needs to be discriminated from a Sinding-Larsen–Johansson lesion. Indirect signs such as hemarthrosis, local tenderness, a palpable gap, and an unusually proximal position of the patella (patella alta) define the injury. Radiographs may look normal if there is only a periosteal degloving without bony involvement. Ultrasound is a quick and safe way to assess periosteal and cartilaginous avulsions. If left untreated the displaced periosteum will continue to form bone and lead to apparent elongation or even duplication of the patella [22]. Avulsion may also occur from the superior and medial margins [23]. Comminuted fractures are rare. They follow a direct fall on the flexed knee and are therefore often open fractures. Transverse stress fractures occur exceptionally either in cerebral palsy and spina bifida patients or in athletes [24]. Anterior knee pain in cerebral palsy patients may also be due to chronic inferior pole fractures with subsequent irritating osseous spurs in the proximal part of the patella tendon [25]. A bipartite patella with an accessory ossicle in the superolateral quadrant should not be confused with a fracture: it is differentiated by its typical localization, its rounded margins, and its usual bilaterality.

Treatment

The pain of significant hemarthrosis is relieved by aspiration. For undisplaced fractures, 4–5 weeks in a cylinder cast with weight-bearing as tolerated is recommended. For displaced fractures the articular surface and the extensor tendon should be reconstructed and fixed by tension-band wiring to prevent osteoarthrosis; functional aftercare is helped by early passive motion [26]. In avulsion fractures the treatment depends on the severity of fragment separation and the amount of bone attached to the avulsed periosteum and cartilage. The surgeon chooses between osteochondral sutures, tension-band wiring, and more rigid types of fixation of larger bone fragments. Pole resection should be avoided [27].

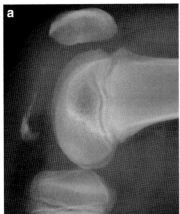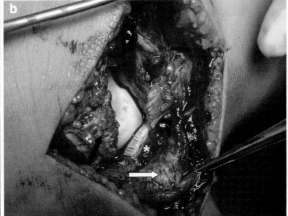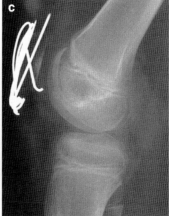

Fig. 12.6 Eleven-year-old boy who jumped from a 2-m wall and sustained a distal patellar sleeve fracture. (**a**) Lateral radiograph: high-lying patella (patella alta)—inferior pole fragments. (**b**) Open reduction: periosteal sleeve (*white arrow*) and inferior pole cartilage (asterisk) opposite cancellous bone of the main patella (*black arrow*). (**c**) Internal fixation with K-wires, tension-band wiring, and osteochondral sutures

Fractures of the Tibial Spine

Mechanism of Injury

The ACL inserts into the medial spine of the proximal tibia. No structure attaches to the lateral spine. Fractures of this tibial eminence are the most common childhood intra-articular fractures of the proximal tibia. Biomechanically they correspond to the ruptured ACL in adults. In children the tibial spine is less resistant to tensile stress than the ACL. However, prior to avulsion of the tibial spine, the ACL stretches due to sequential failure of ligament fibers [28]. A fall from a bicycle with a direct blow on the distal femur with the knee flexed is the most frequently cited cause of injury, followed by hyperextension/rotation trauma sustained during athletic activities (e.g., football or alpine skiing).

Clinical and Radiological Findings

Patients usually present with a painful hemarthrosis and inability to bear weight. Clinically they show a pathological Lachman and anterior drawer test. According to Meyers and McKeevers [29] fractures of the intercondylar eminence can be classified radiologically on a standard lateral view as type I (undisplaced), II (partially displaced, anterior gap but preserved posterior hinge), or III (fully displaced). Zaricznyj [30] suggested an additional type IV for comminuted fractures. Their relative frequency is about 12% (type I), 44% (type II), and 44% (type III) [31–33]. When the physis is still wide open, the whole eminence is avulsed; when it is partially closed, only one of the tubercles may be avulsed. The fragment is usually a single piece with varying amounts of subchondral bone attached, but it may be purely cartilaginous or comminuted. As the fracture often runs through the subchondral plate, the fragment size is easily underestimated on radiograph or even invisible if cartilaginous. Associated injuries to the medial collateral ligament and the menisci (lateral more often than medial) occur mainly with type III fractures but are rare [34]. Arthroscopy may reveal associated injuries, but there seems to be some potential for spontaneous healing as it is rare for non-arthroscoped patients to need secondary operation [35].

Treatment

A painful hemarthrosis is aspirated under sterile conditions. Type I lesions should be immobilized in a cylinder cast for 4 weeks. For type II fractures, closed reduction should be attempted by extending the knee and applying a cylinder cast. Anatomy studies have shown that ACL tension in extension does not prevent fracture reduction [36]. For the failed type II and III lesions, arthroscopic or open reduction is recommended. An interposed meniscal anterior horn and the transverse meniscal ligament are the commonest blocks to reduction and are more likely if the fragment is large. The displaced fragment may be fixed with a trans-epiphyseal suture, wire, wire suture, or crossed retrograde trans-physeal wire according to the surgeon's preference (Fig. 12.7) [31, 37]. The fragment should be anatomically reduced or even countersunk to compensate for the plastic ACL elongation.

Prognosis

A trans-epiphyseal screw may cause a partial growth arrest of the proximal tibial physis [38]. Despite consolidation of the fracture in an anatomical position, chronic anterior instability and loss of full extension are the most frequently reported long-term problems. In 38–70% of patients with a type II or III injury, there was objective evidence (Lachman test, KT 1000 arthrometer) of anterior cruciate laxity. However, only few have subjective complaints if the secondary restraints remain intact [32, 33, 39–41]. It is possible that posttraumatic overgrowth of the tibial spine helps to prevent instability. Obviously the ACL remains elongated with further growth and anatomical reduction does not necessarily prevent ACL laxity. Accordingly, the results of open and closed treatment are similar, provided the fragment consolidates anatomically. Knee laxity does not lead to functional impairment if there is no gross pivot shift. It remains to be seen how functional status and secondary meniscal and osteochondral pathology develop in the long term in posttraumatic lax knees. For the late-presenting patient with a non-united tibial spine associated with pain, giving way, or locking, fixation may still prove successful [42]. Lost extension caused by malunion warrants anatomic fixation if conservative treatment has failed.

Ruptures of the Anterior Cruciate Ligament

Ruptures of the ACL in skeletally immature patients are rare but have become more frequently recognized and reported. The mechanisms of injury are identical to those seen in adults. The site of failure is most commonly at the tibial insertion. Skeletally immature patients with ACL injuries have a narrower intercondylar notch than those with avulsion fractures of the tibial spine [43]. Most patients are male and keen sportsmen involved in contact sport. Thus, they are usually reluctant to consider long periods

Fig. 12.7 Thirteen-year-old boy with a type III avulsion fracture of the ACL. (**a**) Lateral radiograph not conclusive in differentiating between incomplete (type II) and complete (type III) avulsion. (**b**) CT reveals full displacement. (**c** and **d**) Anatomic reduction and wire fixation [28]. Courtesy of Dr. Klaus Parsch, Stuttgart

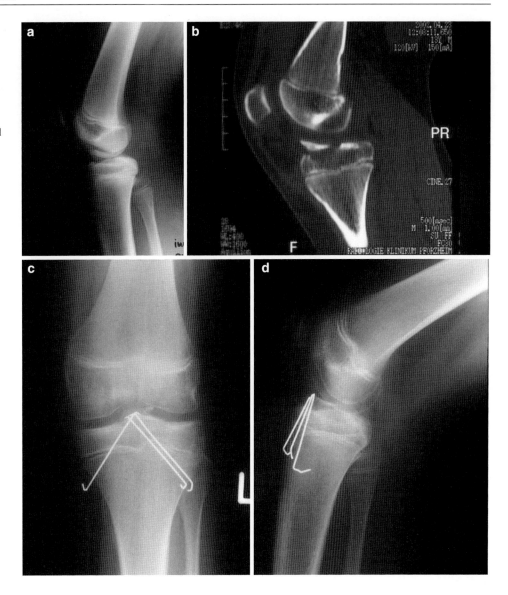

of conservative treatments with physiotherapy, rehabilitation, bracing, and activity modification; they worry about the unpredictable outcome. In addition ACL ruptures during growth are not benign: the natural history is of giving way, pain, and swelling; furthermore, persistent instability may cause meniscal or osteochondral damage.

Treatment

Children generally are highly active and are significantly impaired by ACL rupture. Conservative treatment, direct repair, and extra-articular reconstruction have poor outcomes. Intra-articular reconstruction should be considered when instability prevents participation in sport, conservative treatment has not helped, or if there are associated meniscal or osteochondral injuries [44]. The likelihood of associated meniscal injuries makes primary operative treatment an early

option for many [45, 46]. The gold standard technique of ACL reconstruction in adults, the central one-third bone-patellar-bone graft, may be used in adolescents with only little growth left [47, 48]. Intra-articular reconstruction with a low risk of a growth disturbance is possible if the physis is not damaged [49] or if reconstruction utilizes a soft tissue graft only (e.g., semitendinosus, gracilis, or quadriceps tendon) and is performed through a small diameter tibial drill hole combined with an over-the-top position of the femoral graft. Holes should be drilled perpendicular to the femoral physis or with a physeal-sparing technique (Fig. 12.8) [45].

Prognosis

In patients with an open physis, harvesting of the graft as well as the drill holes may injure the tibial and/or femoral physis with subsequent risk of growth disturbances [50].

Fig. 12.8 Fifteen-year-old soccer player 1 year after arthroscopically assisted replacement of the ACL by a quadriceps tendon graft. The graft fills a trans-epiphyseal tibial drill hole and a physeal-sparing distal femoral canal

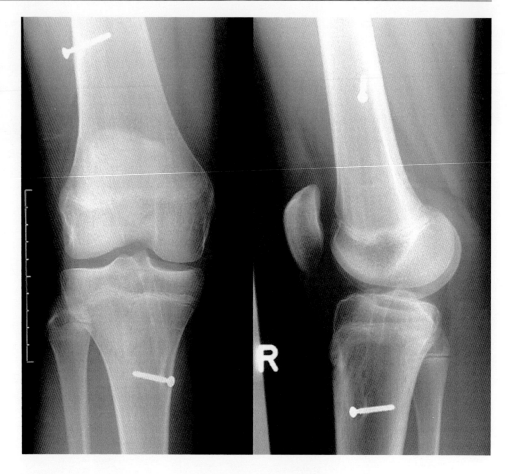

The close anatomic relation of the posterior distal femoral physis and the perichondral ring to the ACL origin has to be considered [51]. Regular review until the end of growth is necessary to detect any axial deviation or leg length discrepancies. Objective and subjective knee stability and re-rupture rates after ACL reconstruction are poorer in children than in adults. This may be attributable to ligamentous laxity during growth and more vigorous sports activities. However, long-term results of knee stability, meniscal degeneration, osteochondral problems, and development of osteoarthritis have so far not been reported.

Intra-articular Physeal Fractures of the Proximal Tibia

Salter–Harris type III, IV and transitional fractures are even rarer than those at the distal femur and, when they do occur, do so in late adolescence. Fracture patterns and treatment are basically the same as for distal intra-articular femoral fractures. Special attention should be paid to associated ligamentous injuries to prevent later instability, osteochondral injuries, as well as meniscal entrapment in the fracture

Fig. 12.9 Fifteen-year-old boy: 20° lack of extension and knee effusion after valgus right knee injury in a fall from a bicycle. (**a**) AP view: possible tibial plateau fracture. (**b**) Repeat radiograph in internal rotation: clear fracture gap. Knee arthroscopy showed meniscus trapped in the gap

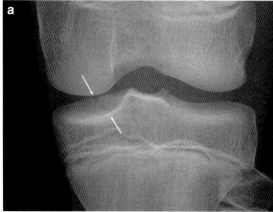
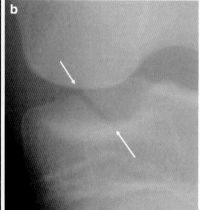

(Fig. 12.9). Arthroscopy helps to assess and fix these fractures.

Avulsion of the Tibial Tuberosity

Mechanism of Injury

This fracture—bony avulsion of the patellar ligament (or tendon), insertion—occurs mainly in adolescent athletes, after either acute forceful contraction of the quadriceps muscle or with acute knee flexion against the contracted quadriceps (e.g., landing after a jump). An association with pre-existing Osgood–Schlatter disease is possible [52]. Bilateral occurrence is reported [53]. Growth disturbances are rare, but in younger patients a genu recurvatum may develop after premature growth arrest [54].

Clinical and Radiological Findings

Patients present with marked pain and a local hematoma over the tuberosity. They are often unable to straight leg raise, to stand, or walk. A high-riding patella is seen with severe displacement and a joint effusion with intra-articular fractures. Severe pain over the anterior lower leg may indicate a compartment syndrome in displaced intra-articular fractures. A lateral radiograph confirms the suspected diagnosis and demonstrates any intra-articular involvement, the size, and displacement of the fragment (which is often much larger than the film suggests). The avulsion fractures of the tibial tuberosity are either extra- or intra-articular (Salter–Harris type III) (Fig. 12.10). The former are regarded as displaced if the tuberosity is elevated more than 5 mm; the latter, as with all intra-articular fractures, if there is a dehiscence or step-off of more than 2 mm. Sleeve avulsion fractures of the patella are well recognized; a similar morphology has been described for the proximal tibia [55]: It is important to be aware of the injury as the patella tendon disrupts with its apophyseal attachment and a sleeve of periosteum. Both may be free of bone and therefore overlooked on the radiograph. The combination of a high-riding patella and local swelling and pain is suspicious. Ultrasound or MRI is the diagnostic investigation of choice. There may be associated injuries like patellar and quadriceps avulsions, meniscal tears, tibial plateau rim fractures, and ligamentous injuries.

Treatment

Undisplaced fracture receives conservative treatment in a cylinder cast for 5–6 weeks. Displaced fractures are treated by open reduction and internal fixation with lag screws performed through a midline vertical incision lateral or medial to the tuberosity (Fig. 12.10). Sometimes an interposed periosteal flap is found under the avulsed fragment. Once this is pulled out, anatomical reduction and fixation of the fragment is easy when the knee is extended. At the end the torn periosteum is sutured over the fracture site. For the isolated bony lesion aftercare is cast free with partial weight-bearing for 6 weeks. If the lesion is an avulsion of the soft tissues (periosteum, patellar ligament) a cylinder cast for 6 weeks provides healing. Consolidation at 6 weeks is confirmed by radiograph. Patients should be followed-up until skeletal maturity.

Epiphysiolysis at the Proximal Tibia

Mechanism of Injury

Separation of the proximal tibial epiphysis (Salter–Harris type I and II fractures) is extremely rare. The tibial tuberosity is part of the proximal tibial epiphysis and will therefore dislocate. The mechanism of injury is an indirect valgus force. Forceful hyperextension with severe anterior displacement of the epiphysis puts the popliteal vessels at risk.

Clinical and Radiological Findings

Signs of circulatory or neurological impairment (peroneal nerve) should be looked for carefully. Undisplaced fractures, mainly simple Salter–Harris type I, may be overlooked if indirect clinical and radiological signs are not considered: pain and swelling over the proximal tibia, an associated fracture of the proximal fibula, and callus formation at the proximal tibia after 4–6 weeks. On the initial radiograph, the angle between the epiphysis and the diaphysis of the tibia should be measured to avoid missing any frontal plane angulation as remodeling is poor.

Treatment

Undisplaced fractures are treated in a long leg plaster cast. Displaced fractures are reduced under anesthesia. The primary goal is to correct any malrotation and angulation in the frontal plane. Only rarely is open reduction necessary and then mainly when soft tissue such as the pes anserinus or periosteum is interposed [56]. Closed or open reduction is stabilized by percutaneous crossed Kirschner-wire pinning and immobilization in a long leg cast for 4–5 weeks.

Radiological follow-up after 8–10 days is recommended; any secondary displacement of up to 20° may be corrected

Fig. 12.10 Fourteen-year-old boy: displaced avulsion fracture of tibial tuberosity with extension into the joint. Anatomic open reduction and internal fixation with two cancellous lag screws. AP (a) and lateral (b) radiographs prior to fixation and after fixations (c) and (d)

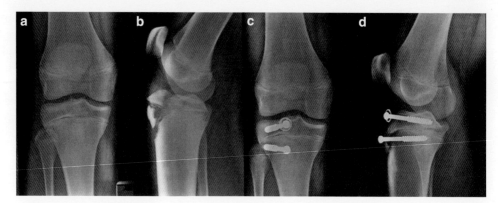

by simple cast wedging. Clinical and radiological review to assess alignment and length should continue 6 monthly for 2 years.

Growth Disturbances

Transient stimulation of the proximal tibial physis with consecutive slight overgrowth of the tibia is the rule but of minor clinical significance. Total or partial growth arrest is rare but may follow even simple Salter–Harris type I or II fractures [57]. It is related to the primary injury and is not preventable: the risk should be discussed with the family before treatment.

Torus Fractures

The compression fractures show no displacement or angulation. They can be treated by immobilization in a long leg plaster for 4–5 weeks. As they are stable, secondary angulation is not a risk. After cast removal consolidation is confirmed clinically by absence of local tenderness. Serial review is unnecessary since growth disturbances do not occur [58].

Bending Fractures of the Proximal Tibia

Mechanism of Injury and Complications

Forces acting upon the lateral aspect of the proximal tibia may either result in a complete metaphyseal fracture of the tibia and fibula or in a partial fracture of the medial cortex of the proximal tibia with or without fibula fracture (greenstick fracture).

The inherent risk of a progressive valgus deformity was first described by Cozen in 1953 [59]. There are two theories to explain post-traumatic valgus deformity:

- Mechanical reasons: entrapment of soft tissues in the fracture gap (periosteum, medial collateral ligament, and the pes anserinus) and loss of medial tethering by avulsion of pes anserinus in combination with ongoing lateral tethering of the intact fibula.
- Asymmetric growth: lack of compression on the fractured medial cortex independent of any interposition leads to a delayed union, a well-known phenomenon in greenstick fractures. The associated and persistent increased local blood supply stimulates the adjacent proximal tibial growth asymmetrically as demonstrated by bone scans [60].

Treatment

Parents must be warned that asymmetric growth may follow this fracture.

Two important and easy steps may prevent the post-traumatic valgus deformity:

1. Recognize even minor valgus deformity on the initial radiograph.
2. Compress the fracture gap at the medial cortex: Under general anesthesia an above-knee cast is applied with the knee in extension and stressed into varus. Patients should be warned further that the cast may slip with the knee extended; after 8 days the cast is wedged. The lateral half of the cast is cut transversely at the level of the fracture and opened with a cast spreader; a spacer is placed into the gap and the cast is completed. This wedging compresses the medially fractured cortex. If the fracture gap can be fully closed valgus deformity can be avoided, while the

tibia will be 5–10 mm longer. Only 4 weeks in plaster is needed. The child should be reviewed for 2 years to detect possible valgus deformity.

If these rules of treatment are not followed significant valgus deformity commonly develops within 1 year of injury (Fig. 12.11) [61]. In children below 5–6 years at injury, the tibia remodels to an S-shaped "serpentine" tibia (proximal tibia in valgus—distal tibia in varus—knee and ankle joint lines parallel) and over the years may grow almost straight [62, 63]. As an alternative to early osteotomy with its inherent risk of deformity recurrence or "wait and see" nihilism in expectation of spontaneous remodeling, hemiepiphysiodesis of the proximal tibia deferred for at least a year after trauma effectively and safely leads to correction within 1 year [64]. Mild rebound valgus deformity after removal occurs in 25% but responds well to re-stapling. The unpredictable further growth and remodeling make it important to review the fracture until skeletal maturity as angular deformity

and tibial overgrowth of up to 10 mm are common (See Chapter 8 of Children's Upper and Lower Limb Orthopaedic Disorders).

Stress Fractures of the Tibia

Pain with weight-bearing (but little night pain) in the absence of trauma, an insidious onset, local tenderness at the proximal tibia in a 10–15-year-old child should make the surgeon suspect a stress fracture. The symptoms may be bilateral. Radiographs may initially be normal, but periosteal reaction and cortical radiolucency at the fracture are visible 2–3 weeks later. A technetium bone scan or an MRI allows early diagnosis. The patient is usually a young athlete, typically a long-distance runner, or has recently changed activity patterns. In girls, one should be alert to the triad of disordered eating, amenorrhea, and osteoporosis. Questions should focus on eating and training habits as well as concomitant symptoms like fatigue, loss of concentration, and cold intolerance.

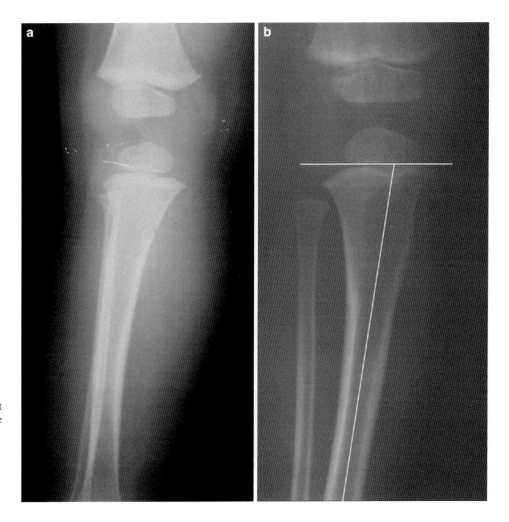

Fig. 12.11 Eighteen-month-old girl with bending fracture of right proximal tibia. (**a**) Bending of the lateral cortex, complete fracture of the medial cortex but no obvious valgus deformity at injury. (**b**) One year later, 12° valgus deformity has developed slowly

Treatment of a stress fracture consists of activity modification, or, if difficult to achieve, a long leg plaster for 3–4 weeks. Preventing recurrence should involve examining the psychosocial environment; liaising with trainers, parents, and teachers; and trying to address all underlying issues such as training hours and intensity, equipment usage, and the pressures placed on the young athlete. When osteoporosis occurs, a team approach with endocrinologist, psychologist, etc., is essential (See Chapter 8).

Diaphyseal Fractures of the Lower Leg

The treatment and prognosis of diaphyseal fractures of the lower leg depend on the bones involved. One should distinguish between tibial fractures with and without an intact fibula: the ratio is about 2:1. Isolated fractures of the fibula are rare and usually due to direct trauma.

Clinical and Radiological Findings

Mild to severe pain and swelling at the fracture site lead to a straightforward clinical diagnosis. With obvious severe deformity which clearly needs reduction, a single radiograph is sufficient to avoid unnecessary positioning in the radiology department. Although disruption of the posterior tibial artery is rare in children with closed fractures, both dorsalis pedis and posterior tibial pulses should be checked clinically and, if absent, by Doppler examination. Unusual severe pain may be the first sign of a compartment syndrome particularly after direct, high-impact, and rollover trauma in adolescents.

Isolated Tibial Fractures

Mechanism of Injury, Fracture Pattern, and Remodeling Capacity

Isolated tibial fractures are the commonest lower limb fracture. They follow indirect rotational forces. They are usually long oblique or spiral fractures at the junction between the middle and the distal thirds, starting anteromedially distally and spiraling up to the proximal postero-lateral cortex. They are seen most often in children below 10 years. Incomplete torus or greenstick fractures account for only about 10% of all tibial fractures. As they are stable they can always be treated conservatively by simple plastering with subsequent wedging to correct minor angular deformities.

In the isolated complete tibial fracture the intact fibula prevents significant shortening, but leads to lateral splinting: While initial tibial angulation rarely exceeds 10°, the more medially directed forces of the posterior flexor muscles cause progressive varus deformity of the tibia in 50%. This usually occurs within 2–3 weeks of injury [65]. Subsequent remodeling is age-dependent: Below 10 years, varus deformities of 10–15° reliably correct themselves. In older children the remodeling capacity is smaller and less predictable. The sagittal plane is the main plane of motion of the adjacent joints. Spontaneous remodeling of up to 20° of recurvatum can be expected in patients younger than 8 years. Procurvatum of the tibia is rare. Rotational deformities (usually external rotation) will persist [66]. They are cosmetically disturbing and, as they are not fully compensated at the knee and ankle, may cause functional impairment if they exceed 10°.

The more pronounced the deformity at consolidation, the longer the remodeling process, and prolonged stimulation of the tibial physis leads to tibial overgrowth of 0.5–1 cm in children under 10 years. In older patients the physis may close prematurely and even result in slight shortening. In summary most initial deformities in the sagittal and frontal plane remodel with time. Nevertheless, one should not accept them if post-traumatic leg length differences are to be avoided [67]. Furthermore, deformities of the tibia are easily visible and cosmetically disturbing due to the lack of medial musculature.

Treatment

Casting is the mainstay of treatment for isolated diaphyseal tibial fractures in children. Even if closed reduction under anesthesia is necessary, the long leg cast can usually be applied as an outpatient. The bimalleolar axis should be compared with the uninjured leg to ensure correct axis and rotation regardless of age. Alignment of the fracture should be monitored 1 week later. If the cast needs to be wedged to correct angulation, this is best performed 8–10 days after injury when the patient is pain free, swelling has subsided, and there is already some fibrous callus (Fig. 12.12). Technically an *open* wedging technique (as described above) is easier, avoids pinching the skin, and carries less risk of increasing compartment pressure:

- Undisplaced or slightly displaced fractures: initially split long leg cast, completed after 4 days and changed 2 weeks after trauma.
- Displaced fractures: closed reduction and posterior long leg split cast which is closed after 4 days. Wedge if greater than 10° deformity at radiological follow-up after 1 week.

Fig. 12.12 Isolated diaphyseal tibial fracture; secondary varus deformity corrected by simple wedging 10 days later

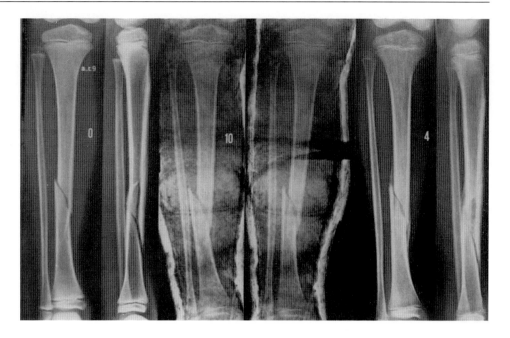

In older children or adolescents with undisplaced fractures a patellar tendon-bearing cast (Sarmiento cast) may be an alternative to allow immediate full weight-bearing [68]. The plaster is removed after 4–5 weeks but re-applied for a further 2–3 weeks if the fracture site is still tender.

• Completely displaced and therefore unstable transverse fractures of the tibia as well as open fractures, patients at risk for a compartment syndrome or poly-traumatized children should be stabilized by intramedullary elastic stable nails [69] or external fixation [70]. Both minimally invasive methods offer short operation times, minimal blood loss, aesthetic scars, preservation of a biologic environment around the fracture site, early mobilization, a low complication rate, and easy metal ware removal. External fixation should be reserved for highly comminuted and/or high-degree open fractures.

Diaphyseal Fractures of Tibia and Fibula

Mechanism of Injury—Remodeling Capacity

These are usually the result of direct trauma to the lower leg (e.g., pedestrian versus car). In contrast to isolated tibial fractures, the muscles of the anterior compartment act as lateral flexors leading to valgus deformity. Spontaneous remodeling should *not* be expected for valgus deformities which should be prevented by proper monitoring during treatment.

Treatment

Basically, stable fractures should be treated conservatively by cast and additional wedging whereas unstable fractures should be stabilized by elastic intramedullary nails or, if these are not available, by external fixation:

• Stable fractures (greenstick fractures, transverse fractures with angulation): after closed reduction split long leg cast which is closed after 4 days. Wedging or new long leg cast if angular deformity at radiological follow-up after 10 days. Non-weight-bearing for 4 weeks followed by a walking cast for another 2 weeks until radiographic consolidation.

• Unstable fractures (fully displaced fractures, oblique fractures with shortening) and polytrauma (Fig. 12.13): stabilization with antegrade descending elastic intramedullary nails or an anteromedial monolateral external fixator [69, 70]. In highly comminuted fractures in adolescents with open growth plates, ring fixation may be a better choice than monolateral fixation which has a significant rate of lost reduction, leading to malunion if not re-manipulated [70].

Prognosis

After open fractures union is usually delayed in younger patients. Patients over 14 years, following both open and closed fractures, show a substantially delayed healing after elastic stable intramedullary nailing (ESIN) [71].

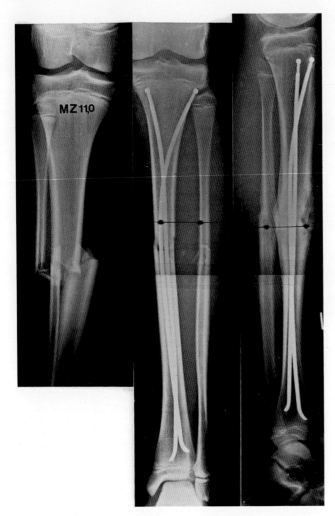

Fig. 12.13 Eleven-year-old boy: unstable diaphyseal fracture of his right tibia and fibula stabilized by antegrade intramedullary flexible nailing. Courtesy of Dr. Klaus Parsch, Stuttgart

Metaphyseal Fractures of the Distal Tibia

As in the proximal tibia, a variety of injury patterns affect the distal metaphysis. Most fractures are incomplete, leaving at least one cortex intact or both impacted.

Torus and Greenstick Fractures

Simple torus fractures (Fig. 12.14) show some recurvatum but no angulation in the frontal plane. True greenstick fractures with impaction of the anterior border and complete fracture of the posterior cortex result in a slight recurvatum. The latter may increase if the deformity is not controlled by applying a below-knee plaster in ankle *plantar flexion* to compress the posterior fracture site. Recurvatum may be combined with valgus deformity and procurvatum with varus [74]. Four weeks in plaster is usually sufficient and bone healing is usually uneventful.

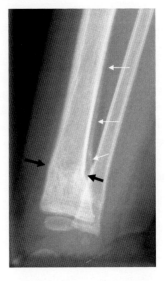

Fig. 12.14 Three-year-old girl with torus fracture (*black arrows*) of her left distal tibia presenting with a history of limping over 4 weeks. Radiographs revealed an old fracture with periosteal reaction along the posterior border of the tibia (*white arrows*). No further action was required

Severe direct impacts, butterfly fragments, age-related borderline indications for ESIN (upper limit at closure of the physis), or technical errors may underlie delayed consolidation or malalignment. The technical principles which need to be considered include adequate nail diameter (usually 2.5–3.5 mm), identical nail diameters, and symmetric prebending of the nails with the maximal curve at the fracture site. Since the tibia is triangular in shape, anatomical stabilization may make it necessary to rotate the nails, sometimes both into valgus if the fibula is intact or vice versa in complete lower leg fractures to counteract the deforming varus forces (isolated tibial facture) or valgus forces (fracture of both tibia and fibula) [72]. Pseudarthrosis after pediatric shaft fractures of the tibia is extremely rare and seen only after high-energy open trauma with or without subsequent osteomyelitis or open reduction followed by unstable fixation [73].

Bending Fractures

Distal bending fractures pose the same problems as those at the proximal tibia, although the subtalar joint may compensate for some mild deformities in the frontal plane. In patients older than 10 years, every malangulation in the frontal plane should be corrected; if not, asymmetric growth stimulation leads to progressive and persistent deformity. In younger patients, spontaneous correction of up to 20° valgus, varus, and recurvatum may be expected. Procurvatum is rare. A below-knee plaster is applied for 4 weeks.

Toddlers' Fractures

These fractures occur in children under 2 years by external rotation of the foot. This causes minimally displaced, short spiral or oblique fractures without fibular involvement. These "toddler fractures" may not be recognized on the initial radiograph but will be discovered at follow-up. It is important that they be considered in the differential diagnosis of limping in otherwise healthy toddlers. Immobilization in a long leg cast for 2–3 weeks sometimes followed by a below-knee cast for 2 weeks is sufficient.

References

1. Sponseller PD, Stanitski CL. Fractures and dislocations about the knee. In: Beaty JH, Kasser JR, eds. Rockwood & Wilkins' Fractures in Children, 5th ed. Philadelphia: Lippincott-Williams & Wilkins; 2001:981–1076.
2. Riseborough EJ, Barrett IR, Shapiro F. Growth disturbances following distal femoral physeal fracture-separations. J Bone Joint Surg Am 1983; 65:885–893.
3. Edmunds I, Nade S. Injuries of the distal femoral growth plate and epiphysis: should open reduction be performed? Aus NZ J Surg 1993; 63:195–199.
4. Lombardo SJ, Harvey JP. Fractures of the distal femoral epiphyses. J Bone Joint Surg Am 1977; 59:742–751.
5. Beaty JH, Kumar A. Fractures about the knee in children. Current concept review. J Bone Joint Surg Am 1994; 76:1870–1880.
6. Czitrom AA, Salter RB, Willis RB. Fractures involving the distal epiphyseal plate of the femur. Int Orthop 1981; 4:269–277.
7. Beck A, Kinzl L, Rüter A, Strecker W. Fractures involving the distal femoral epiphysis. Long-term outcome after completion of growth in primary surgical management. Unfallchirurg 2001; 104:611–616.
8. Eid AM, Hafez MA. Traumatic injuries of the distal femoral physis. Retrospective study on 151 cases. Injury 2002; 33:251–255.
9. Ilharreborde B, Raquillet C, Morel E, et al. Long-term prognosis of Salter-Harris type 2 injuries of the distal femoral physis. J Pediatr Orthop B 2006; 15:433–438.
10. Arkader A, Warner WC Jr, Horn BD, et al. Predicting the outcome of physeal fractures of the distal femur. J Pediatr Orthop 2007; 27:703–708.
11. Stephens DC, Louis E, Louis DS. Traumatic separation of the distal femoral epiphyseal cartilage plate. J Bone Joint Surg Am 1974; 56:1383–1390.
12. Nietos N, Nietosvaara Y, Aalto K, Kallio PE. Acute patellar dislocation in children: Incidence and associated osteochondral fractures. J Pediatr Orthop 1994; 14:513–515.
13. Zaidi A, Babyn P, Astori I, et al. MRI of traumatic patellar dislocation in children. Pediatr Radiol 2006; 36:1163–1170.
14. Nietosvaara Y. The femoral sulcus in children. An ultrasonographic study. J Bone Joint Surg Br 1994; 76:807–809.
15. Yamada Y, Toritsuka Y, Yoshikawa H, et al. Morphological analysis of the femoral trochlea in patients with recurrent dislocation of the patella using three-dimensional computer models. J Bone Joint Surg Br 2007; 89:746–751.
16. Stefancin JJ, Parker RD. First-time traumatic patellar dislocation. Clin Orthop Rel Res 2007; 455:93–101.
17. Nikku R, Nietosvaara Y, Aalto K, Kallio PE. Operative treatment of primary patellar dislocation does not improve medium-term outcome: A 7-year follow-up report and risk analysis of 127 randomized patients. Acta Orthop 2005; 76:699–704.
18. Palmu S, Kallio P, Donell ST, et al. Acute patellar dislocation in children and adolescents: a randomized clinical trial. J Bone Joint Surg Am 2008; 90:463–470.
19. Schillians N, Baltzer AWA, Liebau CH, et al. Osteochondrale Abscherfrakturen bei Kindern. Zentralbl Chir 2001; 126:233–236.
20. Bradley J, Dandy DJ. Osteochondritis dissecans and other lesions of the femoral condyles. J Bone Joint Surg Br 1989; 71:518–522.
21. Dines JS, Fealy S, Potter HG, et al. Outcomes of osteochondral lesions of the knee repaired with a bioabsorbable device. Arthroscopy 2008; 24:62–68.
22. Hunt DM, Somashekar N. A review of sleeve fractures of the patella in children. Knee 2005; 12:3–7.
23. Grogan DP, Carey TP, Leffers D, et al. Avulsion fractures of the patella. J Pediatr Orthop 1990; 10:721–730.
24. Brunner R, Doederlein L. Pathological fractures in patients with cerebral palsy. J Pediatr Orthop 1996; 5:232–238.
25. Senaran H, Holden C, Dabney KW, et al. Anterior knee pain in children with cerebral palsy. J Pediatr Orthop 2007; 27:12–16.
26. Maguire JK, Canale ST. Fractures of the patella in children and adolescents. J Pediatr Orthop 1993; 13:567–571.
27. Kastelec M, Veselko M. Inferior patellar pole avulsion fractures: osteosynthesis compared with pole resection. J Bone Joint Surg Am 2004; 86:696–701.
28. Noyes FR, Delucas JL, Torvik PJ. Biomechanics of anterior cruciate ligament failure: an analysis of strain-rate sensitivity and mechanisms of failure in primates. J Bone Joint Surg 1974; 56-A:236–253.
29. Meyers MH, McKeever FM. Fracture of the intercondylar eminence of the tibia. J Bone Joint Surg 1959; 41-A:209–220.
30. Zaricznyj B. Avulsion fracture of the tibial eminence: treatment by open reduction and pinning. J Bone Joint Surg Am 1977; 59:1111–1114.
31. Grönkvist H, Hirsch G, Johansson L. Fracture of the anterior tibial spine in children. J Pediatr Orthop 1984; 4:465–468.
32. Janarv PM, Westblad P, Johansson C, et al. Long-Term Follow-up of anterior tibial spine fractures in children. J Pediatr Orthop 1995; 15:63–68.
33. Willis RB, Blokker C, Stoll TM, et al. Long-term follow-up of anterior tibial eminence fractures. J Pediatr Orthop 1993; 13:361–364.
34. Ishibashi Y, Tsuda E, Sasaki T, et al. Magnetic resonance imaging aids in detecting concomitant injuries in patients with tibial spine fractures. Clin Orthop Rel Res 2005; 434:207–212.
35. Molander ML, Wallin G, Wikstad I. Fracture of the intercondylar eminence of the tibia. J Bone Joint Surg Br 1981; 63:89–91.
36. Hallam PJB, Fazal MA, Ashwood N, et al. An alternative to fixation of displaced fractures of the anterior intercondylar eminence in children. J Bone Joint Surg 2002; 84-B:579–582.
37. Mauch F, Parsch K. Internal fixation of intercondylar eminence avulsion in children. Operat Orthop Traumatol 2004; 16:418–432.
38. Mylle J, Reynders P, Broos P. Transepiphyseal fixation of anterior cruciate avulsion in a child. Report of a complication and review of the literature. Arch Orthop Trauma Surg 1993; 112:101–103.

39. Baxter MP, Wiley JJ. Fractures of the tibial spine in children. An evaluation of knee stability. J Bone Joint Surg 1988; 70-B:228–230.

40. Kocher MS, Foreman ES, Micheli LJ. Laxity and functional outcome after arthroscopic reduction and internal fixation of displaced tibial spine fracture in children. Arthroscopy 2003; 19:1085–1090.

41. Smith JB. Knee instability after fractures of the intercondylar eminence of the tibia. J Pediatric Orthop 1984; 4:462–464.

42. Kawate K, Fujisawa Y, Yajima H, et al. Seventeen-year follow-up of a reattachment of a nonunited anterior tibial spine avulsion fracture. Arthroscopy 2005; 21:760.

43. Kocher MS, Mandiga R, Klingele K, et al. Anterior cruciate ligament injury versus tibial spine fracture in the skeletally immature knee: a comparison of skeletal maturation and notch width index. J Pediatr Orthop 2004; 24:185–188.

44. Janarv PM, Nyström A, Werner S, Hirsch G. Anterior cruciate ligament injuries in skeletally immature patients. J Pediatr Orthop 1996; 16:673–677.

45. Aichroth PM, Patel DV, Zorilla P. The natural history and treatment of rupture of the anterior cruciate ligament in children and adolescents. J Bone Joint Surg Br 2002; 84:38–41.

46. Arbes St, Resinger C, Vécsei V, et al. The functional outcome of total tears of the anterior cruciate ligament (ACL) in the skeletally immature patient. Int Orthop 2007; 31:471–475.

47. Kannus P, Järvinen M. Knee ligament injuries in adolescents. J Bone Joint Surg Br 1988; 70:772–776.

48. McCarroll JR, Shelbourne KD, Porter DA, et al. Patellar tendon graft reconstruction for midsubstance anterior cruciate ligament rupture in junior high school athletes. Am J Sports Med 1994; 22:478–484.

49. Nakhostine M, Bollen SR, Cross MJ. Reconstruction of midsubstance anterior cruciate rupture in adolescents with open physis. J Pediatr Orthop 1995; 15:286–287.

50. Kocher MS, Saxon HS, Hovis WD, et al. Management and complications of anterior cruciate ligament injuries in skeletally immature patients: a survey of the Herodicus Society and The ACL Study group. J Pediatr Orthop 2002; 22:452–457.

51. Kocher MS, Hovis WD, Curtin MJ, et al. Anterior cruciate ligament reconstruction in skeletally immature knees: an anatomical study. Am J Orthop 2005; 34:285–290.

52. Ogden JA, Tross RB, Murphy MJ. Fractures of the tibial tuberosity in adolescents. J Bone Joint Surg Am 1980; 62:205–215.

53. Neugebauer A, Muensterer OJ, Buehligen U, Till H. Bilateral avulsion fractures of the tibial tuberosity: a double case for open reduction and fixation. Eur J Trauma Emerg Surg 2008; 34:83–87.

54. Christie MJ, Dvonch VM. Tibial tuberosity avulsion fracture in adolescents. J Pediatr Orthop 1981; 1:391–394.

55. Davidson D, Letts M. Partial sleeve fractures of the tibia in children: an unusual fracture pattern. J Pediatr Orthop 2002; 22:36–40.

56. Harries TJ, Lichtmann DM, Lonon WD. Irreducible Salter Harris II fracture of the proximal tibia. J Pediatr Orthop 1983; 3:92–95.

57. Burkhart SS, Peterson HA. Fractures of the proximal tibial epiphysis. J Bone Joint Surg Am 1979; 61:996–1002.

58. Von Laer L, Jani L, Cuny T, et al. The proximal fracture of the lower leg in adolescence. Cause and prophylaxis of the posttraumatic genu valgum. Unfallheilkunde 1982; 85:215–225.

59. Cozen L. Fracture of proximal portion of tibia in children followed by valgus deformity. Surg Gyn Obstet 1953; 97:183–188.

60. Zionts LE, Harcke HAT, Brooks KM, et al. Post-traumatic tibia valga: a case demonstrating asymmetric activity at the proximal growth plate on technetium bone scan. J Pediatr Orthop 1977; 7:458–462.

61. Parsch K, Manner G, Dippe K. Genu valgum nach proximaler Tibiafraktur beim Kind. Arch Orthop Unfall-Chir 1977; 90:289–297.

62. Brammar TJ, Rooker GD. Remodeling of valgus deformity secondary to proximal metaphyseal fracture of the tibia. Injury 1998; 29:558–560.

63. Tuten R, Keeler KA, Gabos PG, et al. Posttraumatic tibia valga in children. A long-term follow-up note. J Bone Joint Surg Am 1999; 81:799–810.

64. Stevens PM, Pease F. Hemiepiphysiodesis for posttraumatic tibial valgus. J Pediatr Orthop 2006; 26:385–392.

65. Teitz CC, Carter DR, Frankel VH. Problems associated with tibial fractures with intact fibulae. J Bone Joint Surg Am 1980; 62:770–776.

66. Shannak AO. Tibial fractures in children: a follow-up study. J Pediatr Orthop 1988; 8:306–310.

67. Von Laer L, Kaelin L, Girard T. Late results following shaft fractures of the lower extremities in the growth period. Z Unfallchir Versicherungsmed Berufskr 1989; 82:209–215.

68. Austin RT. The Sarmiento tibial plaster: a prospective study of 145 fractures. Injury 1981; 13:10–22.

69. Ligier JN, Metaizeau JP, Prevot J, et al. Elastic stable intramedullary nailing of femoral shaft fractures in children. J Bone Joint Surg Br 1988; 70:74–77.

70. Gordon JE, Schoenecker PL, Oda JE, et al. A comparison of monolateral and circular external fixation of unstable diaphyseal tibial fractures in children. J Pediatr Orthop B 2003; 12:338–345.

71. Gordon JE, Gregush RV, Schoenecker PL, et al. Complications after titanium elastic nailing of pediatric tibial fractures. J Pediatr Orthop 2007; 27:442–446.

72. Lascombes P, Haumont T, Journeau P. Use and abuse of flexible intramedullary nailing in children and adolescents. J Pediatr Orthop 2006; 26(6):827–834.

73. Lewallen RP, Peterson HA. Nonunion of long bone fractures in children: a review of 30 cases. J Pediatr Orthop 1985; 5:135–142.

74. Domzalski ME, Lipton GE, Lee D, et al. Fractures of the distal tibial metaphysis in children. Patterns of injury and results of treatment. J Pediatr Orthop 2006; 26:171–176.

Chapter 13

Ankle Fractures

Klaus Parsch and Francisco Fernandez Fernandez

Incidence and Mechanism of Injury

Injuries of the ankle joint are common. According to Peterson [1] physeal injuries of the distal tibia and fibula account for 25% of all physeal fractures. About 60% of physeal ankle fractures occur during sports activities and are more common in males than in females [2]. In his monograph Poland [3] pointed out that children's ligaments are stronger than physeal cartilage. Where adults would sustain ligamentous injuries the same forces will cause fractures of the physis in children.

Classification

After Poland [3] and Aitken [4], Salter and Harris coined a classification for physeal injuries in the ankle joint (Fig. 13.1) [5].

The classification of physeal injuries in the distal tibia and fibula of Dias and Tachdjian follows the injury mechanism shown in Fig. 13.2 [6].

Treatment

General Aspects

Non-displaced fractures can be simply immobilized in a cast. Displaced fractures can be treated by closed reduction and cast immobilization. If closed reduction cannot be *maintained* internal fixation is necessary. If closed reduction is

K. Parsch (✉)
Orthopaedic Department, Pediatric Olgahospital, Stuttgart, Germany

not possible, open reduction and internal fixation are indicated. The anatomic type of the fracture defined by the Salter and Harris (SH) classification, the mechanism of injury following Dias and Tachdjian, and the amount of displacement, especially the intraarticular lesion, must be considered. The status of the skin and the neurovascular function/integrity may require emergency treatment in some cases.

Salter and Harris Type I

These are rare injuries. The majority will have some metaphyseal fragments discovered classifying them SH type II. True displaced SH type I lesions should be reduced as an emergency for protection of the soft tissues and the skin. Complete reduction may be possible by closed means; if not open reduction and crossed K-wire fixation are indicated. Immobilization for 4 weeks in a non-weight bearing above-knee cast is followed by a weight bearing one for another 3 weeks [7].

Salter and Harris Type II

SH type II fractures can be undisplaced or displaced. The majority result from a pronation-eversion mechanism, but some have the supination-inversion mechanism [6]. SH type II fractures are the most common injuries [2].

Treatment

We treat *non-displaced fractures* with a below-knee cast for 3 weeks, followed by a short walking cast for another 3 weeks. Some prefer to use a long above-knee cast initially [2].

Displaced SH type II fractures should be reduced. We recommend a closed reduction under general anesthesia. If that is successful an above-knee cast should be applied.

139

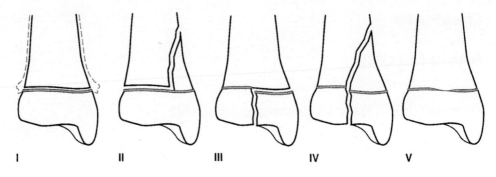

Fig. 13.1 Classification of Salter and Harris. I: Separation of the distal tibial metaphysis from the epiphysis; II: Separation of the distal tibia with metaphyseal fragment; III: Intraepiphyseal fracture of the distal tibia; IV: Fracture separation of distal tibial meta- and epiphysis; V: Crush injury of the distal tibial physis. From Cummings [7]. Used with permission

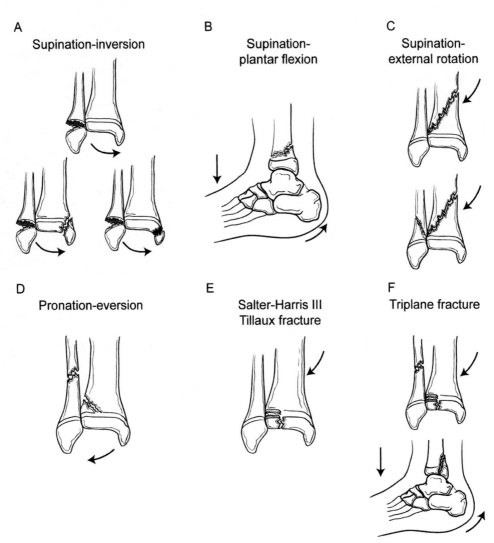

Fig. 13.2 Classification of Dias and Tachdjian. (**A**) *Supination-inversion:* Grade 1 adduction force causes avulsion of the distal fibular epiphysis, while grade 2 with further inversion produces additional Salter–Harris IV or III injury of the distal medial tibia. (**B**) *Supination-plantar flexion:* The plantarflexion forces displace the tibial epiphysis directly posteriorly producing a Salter–Harris I or II lesion. (**C**) *Supination-external rotation:* In grade I the external rotation forces result in a Salter–Harris II fracture. The distal fragment is displaced posteriorly. In grade II with more external rotation a spiral fracture of the distal tibia is produced. (**D**) *Pronation-eversion external rotation* forces cause a distal fibular fracture and a distal tibial fragment displaced later- ally and possibly a lateral or posterolateral Thurston Holland fragment. (**E**) *Juvenile Tillaux fracture:* Salter–Harris III fracture involving the anterolateral part of the distal tibia. (**F**) *Triplane fracture* is produced by a combination of external rotation and plantar flexion forces. The fracture consists of three major fragments: the anterolateral quadrant of the distal tibial epiphysis, the medial and posterior portions of the epiphysis, and the tibial metaphysis. Triplane fractures can have two parts, three, or even four parts. Triplane fractures have the appearance of a Salter–Harris type III on the AP radiograph and of a Salter–Harris type II fracture on the lateral view. From Dias and Tachdjian [6]. Used with permission

Fig. 13.3 Fifteen-year-old boy after trampoline accident with pronation external rotation injury. (**a**) AP view of Salter–Harris II injury and distal fracture of fibula. (**b**) AP view after unsuccessful attempt at closed reduction. (**c**) AP view after open reduction, infolding of periosteal entrapment. (**d**) AP view after 4 months. Anatomic healing of tibia

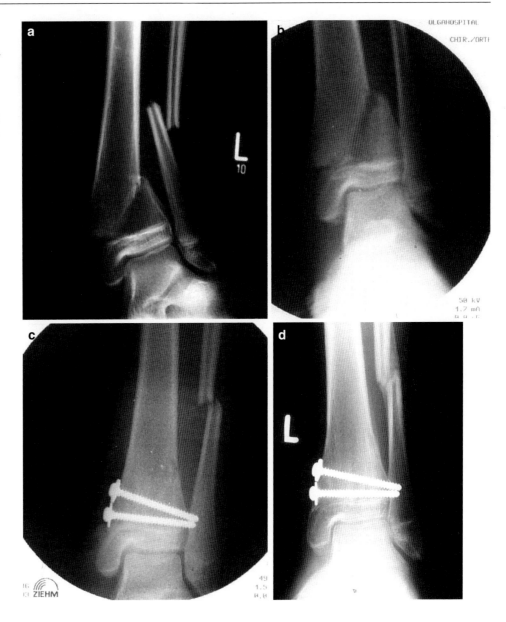

There is controversy as to how much residual displacement should acceptable after closed reduction. If the fracture gap is more than 2 mm, periosteum may be trapped and one should proceed to open reduction followed by internal fixation (Fig. 13.3).

Premature Physeal Closure

Wirth et al. [8] showed in their experimental studies on sheep that implantation of periosteum resulted in inhibition of longitudinal growth and the formation of bony bridges. Ablation of physeal cartilage combined with periosteal insertion results in dramatic injury that cannot be corrected [9]. Barmada et al. [10] noted the importance of entrapped periosteum causing a gap. If a residual gap is not closed the

incidence of premature physeal closure (PPC) is increased to 60%, while the incidence decreased to 17% in those where no gap was present. Anatomic reduction must be achieved at all costs to decrease the risk of PPC [11].

Our Preferred Method

In SH type II fractures with displacement we recommend closed reduction under general anesthesia. The patient must be fully relaxed to allow the reduction manoeuvre, which will be noticed by a palpable click which can also be heard. Complete reduction should be confirmed on the image intensifier. Radiographic documentation is advised in two planes. The patient is immobilized in an above-knee long leg cast for 3 weeks followed by a short walking cast for another 3 weeks.

If complete reduction is not achieved, as revealed on the image intensifier, during the same anesthesia we proceed to open reduction. As soon as the entrapped periosteum is anatomical reduction is easy most of the time. The metaphyseal fragment is fixed by one or two screws inserted horizontally to provide a stable retention of the fragments (Fig. 13.3). As an alternative crossed K-wires can be used (Fig. 13.4). Postoperative immobilization is achieved by a below-knee cast for 3 weeks, followed by a below-knee walking cast for another 3 weeks.

If the rules concerning non-acceptance of incomplete reduction caused by periosteal entrapment are followed, SH type II fractures are a benign lesion and the outcome will be satisfactory. If a gap of more than 2 mm persists, there is a high risk of PCC [10].

Salter–Harris Types III and IV

Types III and IV distal tibial epiphyseal fracture are very demanding. The most frequent one is after supination-inversion injury. As described by Dias and Tachdjian [6] lesser supination force will cause a distal fibular epiphyseal avulsion, while stronger deforming forces will cause an

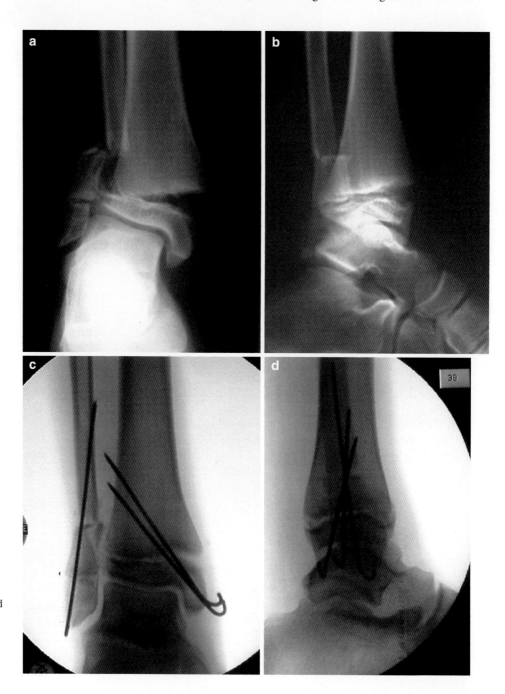

Fig. 13.4 Fifteen-year-old female athlete after pronation-eversion trauma playing soccer. (**a**) AP view of Salter–Harris II lesion and distal fibular fracture. (**b**) Lateral view of Salter–Harris II fracture with gapping. (**c**) AP view after closed reduction which was not stable. Crossed Kirschner wires provide stable fixation. (**d**) Lateral view after percutaneous pinning of Salter–Harris II fracture

avulsion of the medial malleolus, rarely type III (intraepiphyseal), more frequently type IV including a metaphyseal fragment.

Treatment

Anatomic reduction is necessary in to avoid, if possible, premature physeal closure. Even with a near perfect reduction small fragments from local crush injury can cause partial growth arrest. The age of the child is important: the young child will have a higher risk than the more mature patient shortly before the physes close. All type III and IV injuries must be followed for at least 2 years after injury in order to recognize any physeal damage followed by growth arrest in the young patients until maturity.

Undisplaced type III and IV lesions can be treated conservatively. This treatment is indicated only if the gap is 1 mm or less. Some prefer a computed tomography (CT) scan before initiating conservative treatment and also for control in the cast [7]. One must be sure that a close follow-up is guaranteed with review at 2, 4, and 6 weeks after injury. Secondary displacement can occur inside a cast as soon as posttraumatic swelling of the ankle has subsided. Immobilization time is 4 weeks in an above-knee cast followed by 3 weeks in a below-knee walking cast. Clinical and possibly radiological controls are obligatory for at least 2 years after the trauma, so that PCC is not overlooked (Fig. 13.5).

Displaced type III and type IV injuries must be correctly diagnosed by radiographs in two planes; oblique radiographs may be helpful to obtain a correct diagnosis. If available CT scan or magnetic resonance imaging (MRI) can contribute to an exact diagnosis similar to imaging in triplane fractures [12].

Surgical treatment is indicated in all displaced type III and IV lesions with more than 1 mm gap. Big epi-metaphyseal fragments have to be reduced anatomically. After provisional coaption with one or two K-wires the fragments are fixed by two transverse screws. The diameter of the intraepiphyseal screw must be according to the size of the epiphysis and should not interfere with the growth plate, while the metaphyseal screw can be larger (Fig. 13.6).

In younger children with small fragments several K-wires can be used in an attempt to fix the pieces of bone and cartilage in their anatomic position. If the fibular physis is displaced a longitudinal K-wire will help retain that part of the problem. The young children with a severe crush of the medial malleolus plus adjacent metaphysis carries a high risk of PPC, even if seemingly anatomical reduction is achieved. Follow-up reviews are mandatory until maturity, in order to recognize and treat the dreaded medial growth arrest causing deformity (Fig. 13.7). If medial growth arrest causes varus deformity, supramalleolar corrective osteotomy is indicated (Fig. 13.8).

Transitional Fractures

An asymmetric pattern of closure of the distal tibial physis during the last 18 months produces a special fracture pattern not seen in younger patients, where the physes are still wide open. This group of fractures has been labeled transitional fractures because they occur during the transition from

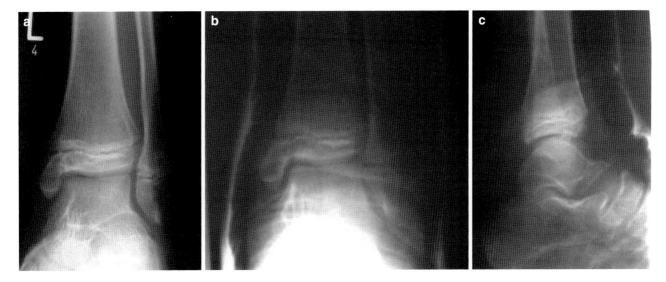

Fig. 13.5 Twelve-year-old boy after supination inversion injury playing football. (a) AP radiograph of non-displaced Salter–Harris III fracture. (b) AP view, after conservative treatment and immobilization in a below-knee cast. (c) Lateral view of undisplaced fracture in the cast

Fig. 13.6 Eleven-year-old girl had fallen from a horse with supination-inversion trauma. (**a**) Displaced Salter–Harris IV fracture seen on an oblique view of the ankle joint. Impaction trauma on the medial dome of talus. (**b**) AP and lateral view after open reduction, fixation with two transverse screws. (**c**) AP radiograph at age 15, 4 years post–trauma, showing anotomical (**d**) Lateral view at age 15, 4 years posttrauma

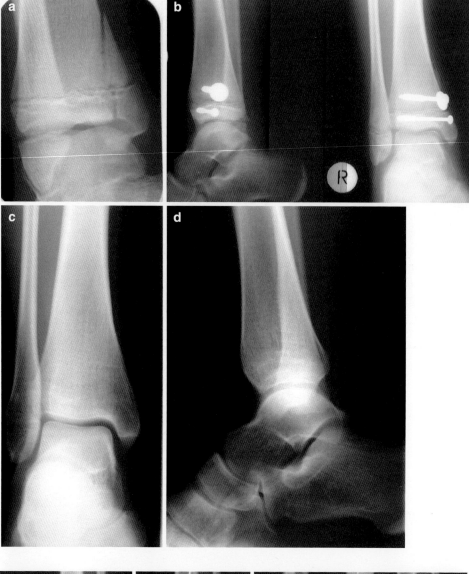

Fig. 13.7 Fifteen-year-old female athlete with severe supination inversion injury. (**a**) AP view of Salter–Harris IV fracture dislocation. Complete displacement of medial malleolus. (**b**) AP view after tension-band osteosynthesis of the medial malleolus and fibula. (**c**) Ankle joint in two planes 16 months later

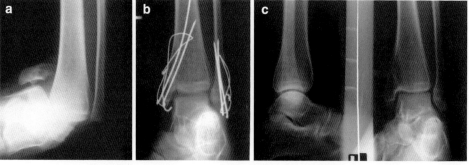

a skeletally immature to a skeletally mature ankle. There is the SH type III *Tillaux fracture* and a variety of triplane fractures. While the Tillaux fracture type was described for adults in the late nineteenth century [13] the triplane fractures were identified as a separate entity in the late twentieth century by Marmor [14] and Lynn [15]. They seem to be caused by external rotation, with stage I causing Tillaux fractures and further external rotation triplane fractures, while grade II will cause additional fracture of the distal fibula [16].

Fig. 13.8 Nine-year-old girl who had fallen off a ladder. (**a**) AP view of Salter–Harris IV with medial crush zone. (**b**) AP view after open reduction and K-wire fixation. (**c**) AP view 6 years later with medial growth arrest and varus deformity. (**d**) AP view at $16\frac{1}{2}$ years, 1 year after supramalleolar corrective osteotomy using a medial bone graft

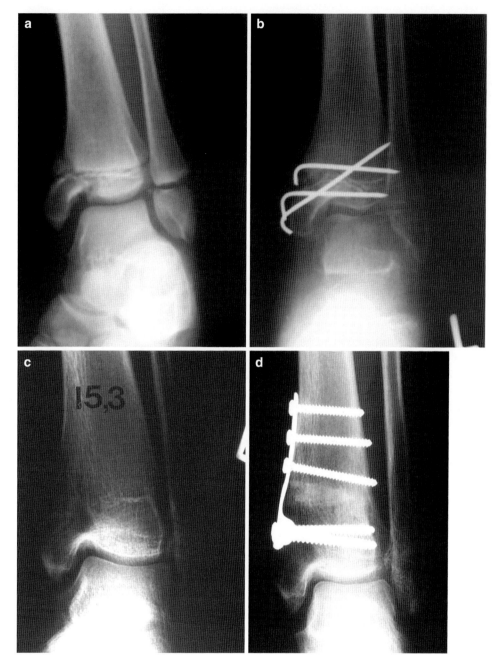

Tillaux Fracture

This SH type III fracture occurs with external rotation of the foot. The anteroinferior tibiofibular ligament through its attachment avulses an anterolateral fragment of the tibial physis. The position of the fibula prevents major displacement of the Tillaux fragment. Clinically local tenderness and swelling is present at the anterolateral aspect of the joint. In uncertain cases, when anteroposterior (AP) radiograph is not clear, an oblique view of the ankle joint will be helpful. If available, CT scan or MRI will show the fracture line clearly [12].

Treatment

For Tillaux fractures which are undisplaced or have a gap of less than 2 mm, we immobilize the patient in a below-knee cast with the ankle joint in neutral dorsiflexion. Secondary

Fig. 13.9 Fifteen-year-old girl after external rotation trauma during track event. (**a**) AP radiograph of displaced Tillaux fracture. (**b**) CT scan reveals a two-part distal tibial fracture fracture with two fragments. (**c**) AP radiograph after open reduction and insertion of cannulated screw

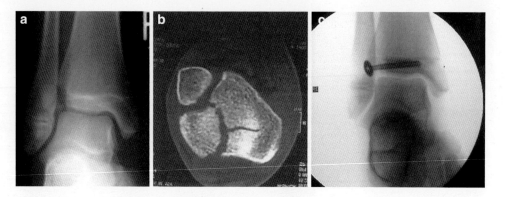

displacement is possible, CT controls after a few days are indicated, as on plain film control a change might not be noted. So CT scans are indicated after a few days as any displacement may not be seen radiographically.

Displacement of over 2 mm should be reduced and fixed. This can be done by a percutaneous cannulated screw. A percutaneous Kirschner wire will help to manipulate the fracture into its anatomical position. The screw has its diameter according to the size of the physis and should be inserted horizontally, parallel to the growth plate. If closed reduction is not possible, open reduction is performed through a small anterolateral incision, followed by the insertion of a lag screw inside the physis, parallel to the growth plate (Fig. 13.9). The intraarticular fragment can be fixed arthroscopically [17, 18].

Prognosis of reduced and fixed Tillaux fractures is good as long as the articular surface has been restored. Premature physeal closure is not a problem, because this fracture occurs only in patients who are about to close their physis.

Triplane Fracture

Marmor [14] described an irreducible ankle fracture in a child that at operation consisted of three fragments. Lynn [15] reported on two additional cases and coined the name triplane fracture.

Triplane fracture may consist of two parts, a large posterolateral epiphyseal fragment with its posterior metaphyseal fragment attached to it.

It may consist of three parts with a large epiphyseal fragment and its metaphyseal component. In addition there is a smaller anterolateral epiphyseal fragment.

In the four-part lateral triplane fracture there is an anterior split of the epiphyseal fragment into two, while the posterior fragment is the larger one with its metaphyseal component attached to it.

Intramalleolar triplane fracture as described by von Laer [19] is a rare extraarticular variant [20, 21] of the standard intraarticular triplane fracture.

Triplane fractures occur most frequently in adolescents, the main cause being sports injuries. Swelling and pain are

more on the lateral aspect of the ankle joint and because of the fixed fibula there is no major visible deformity in these injuries.

Radiography in the AP plane does show the intraepiphyseal fracture line, while the metaphyseal segment of the fracture is better seen on the lateral plane radiograph. Oblique views are helpful, if other imaging methods are not available. While most acute distal tibial fractures can be well diagnosed by plain radiographs, the complex status of intraarticular damage is better diagnosed with the help of a CT scan or MRI [22].

CT scans are recommended in suspected triplane fracture, in order to identify the intraepiphyseal and intraarticular situation [19, 23]. MRI is an ideal tool to identify epi- and metaphyseal injury as well as the damage to the soft tissues [12]. MRI can visualize entrapped periosteum from the metaphyseal fragment, which can be a major obstacle to closed reduction.

Treatment

Undisplaced triplane fractures with a gap smaller than 2 mm and extraarticular type D fractures can be treated with a below-knee cast in neutral position. Immobilization is 3 weeks in a long leg cast without weight bearing followed by another 3 weeks in a weight bearing below-knee cast.

Any intraarticular displacement of more than 2 mm needs surgical reduction. Preoperative CT scans provide a clear picture and shows whether one is treating a two- three- or four-segmented triplane tibial epiphyseolysis (TPE) [24]. The three-segmented type is well described by the "Mercedes star" [25].

Surgical reduction in two-segment TPE is done by an anteromedial incision. The fracture site is irrigated to remove debris. Most often entrapped periosteum has to be removed in order to be able to reduce the metaphyseal segment which will allow easier reduction of the intraepiphyseal lesion. A second anterolateral incision is sometimes needed for removal of the interposed periosteum. The reduced fracture is stabilised by provisional K-wires. Satisfactory reduction

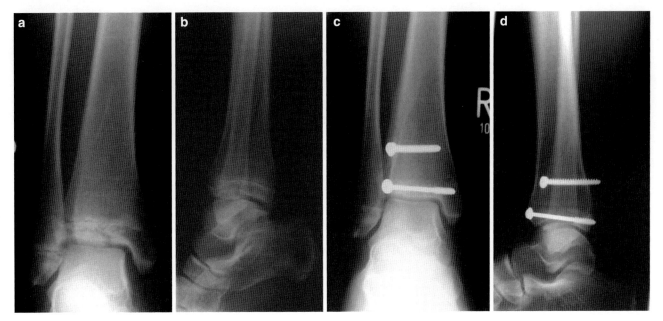

Fig. 13.10 Thirteen-year-old girl after fall from her bicycle with eversion trauma. (**a**) AP radiograph of two-part triplane fracture with 4 mm intraarticular gap. (**b**) Lateral view of the fracture shows displacement within the joint. (**c**) AP view after open reduction, removal of periosteum entrapment, and fixation with an epiphyseal and metaphyseal screws. (**d**) Lateral view with complete closure of the intraarticular fracture gap inside the joint

must be controlled on the image intensifier in both planes. Two cancellous screws are inserted horizontally from medial to lateral, or from anterior to posterior depending on the fracture pattern (Fig. 13.10).

Arthroscopy-assisted reduction and percutaneous fixation are described for triplane fractures (Fig. 13.11), at least taking care of the intraarticular part of that injury. The published data are small series or single case reports [17, 18, 26, 27].

Immobilization after surgical reduction, open or arthroscopically assisted, is needed for a 6-week period in a below-knee cast, the first 3 weeks without and the second 3 weeks with weight bearing.

The outcome after surgical treatment of triplane fractures is satisfactory as long as anatomical reduction of the intraepiphyseal and intraarticular lesion has been complete (Fig. 13.12). If steps of more than 2 mm are left behind osteoarthrosis will develop later.

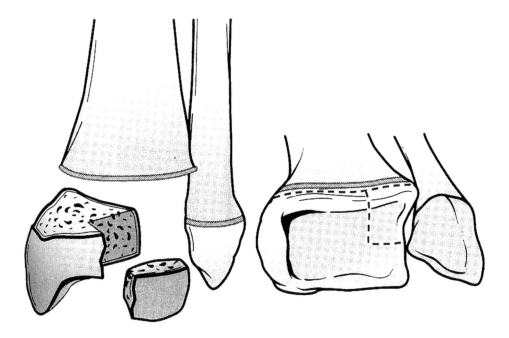

Fig. 13.11 Three-part triplane fracture. From Cummings [7]. Used with permission

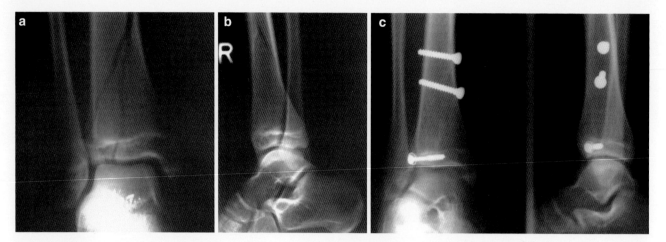

Fig. 13.12 Thirteen-year-old girl who fell during volleyball game. (**a**) AP view of triplane fracture (three fragments). (**b**) Lateral view of triplane fracture. (**c**) AP and lateral view 4 months after open reduction and fixation with one epiphyseal screw and two metaphyseal screws

Lateral Ankle Sprain

Sprained ankles are common lesions. After a phase of surgical treatment of ligamentous injuries of the ankle in the past it became obvious that conservative treatment achieved the same good results. It is widely accepted today that purely ligamentous injuries are treated with in 3 weeks a below-knee walking cast. Sprained ankles with an avulsed fragment of the distal fibula are a separate entity and need active treatment [28].

Avulsion Fractures of the Distal Fibula

Avulsion fractures of the distal fibula rarely occur in young children, but may be seen occasionally in adolescents, where ankle sprains are more common. Radiographic identification is not always obvious and sometimes needs a close-up view and a special technique [29].

Treatment

Radiologically visible fragments are avulsions from the distal fibula. The avulsed fragments are fixed with two Kirschner wires in younger patients (Fig. 13.13), and with a

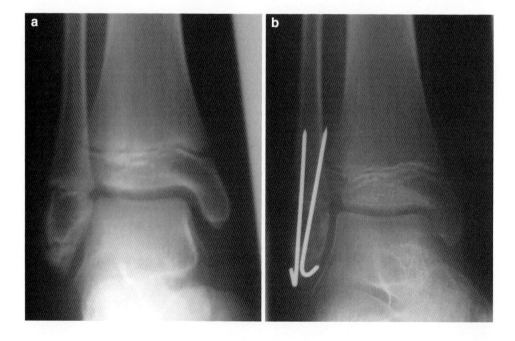

Fig. 13.13 Twelve-year-old female volleyball player injured during game. (**a**) Distal fibular fracture, not yet displaced. (**b**) AP view after fixation with two K-wires buried under the skin

screw in the almost mature adolescents. If these fragments are not recognized they may cause chronic pain, less frequently instability. In a small series of adolescent athletes, removal of a bony fragment gave relief from pain. The symptoms seemed to have come more from the bony fragment than from the ligamentous injury [30, 31].

References

1. Peterson HA, Madhog R, Benson JT, et al. Physeal fractures: Part 1. Epidemiology in Olmsted County Minnesota. J Pediatr Orthop 1994; 14: 423–430.
2. Spiegel PG, Cooperman DR, Laros GS. Epiphyseal fractures of the distal ends of the tibia and fibula. J Bone Joint Surg Am 1978; 60: 1046–1050.
3. Poland J. Traumatic separation of the epiphysis. Smith, Elder and Co, 1898 (Portions reprinted). Clin Orthop Relat Res 1965; 41: 7–18.
4. Aitken AP. The end result of the fractured distal tibial epiphysis. J Bone Joint Surg 1936; 18: 685–691.
5. Salter RB, Harris WB. Injuries involving the epiphyseal plate. J Bone Joint Surg Am 1963; 45: 587–622
6. Dias LS, Tachdjian MO Physeal injuries of the ankle in children. Clin Orthop Relat Res 1978; 136: 230–233.
7. Cummings RJ. Distal tibial and fibular fractures. In: Beaty JH, Kasser JH, eds. Rockwood and Wilkins' Fractures in Children 6th ed. Philadelphia: Lippincott Williams and Wilkins; 2001: 1077–1128.
8. Wirth T, Byers S, Byard RW, et al. The implantation of cartilaginous and periostal tissue into growth plate defects. Intern Orthop (SICOT) 1994; 18: 220–228.
9. Gruber HE, Phieffer LS, Wattenbarger JW. Physeal fractures, Part II: Fate of interposed periostium in a physeal fracture. J Pediatr Orthop 2002; 22: 710–716.
10. Barmada A, Gyanor TP, Mubarak SJ. Premature physeal closure following distal tibia physeal fractures. A new radiographic predictor. J Pediatr Orthop 2003; 23: 733–739.
11. Rohmiller MT, Gaynor TP, Pawalek J, et al. Salter-Harris I and II fractures of the distal tibia: Does mechanism of injury relate to premature physeal closure? J Pediatr Orthop 2006; 26: 322–328.
12. Seifert J, Matthes G, Hinz P, et al. Role of magnetic resonance imaging in the diagnosis of distal tibia fractures in adolescents. J Pediatr Orthop 2003; 23: 727–732.
13. Tillaux PJ. Traite d'anatomie topographique avec applications à la chirurgie, 2nd ed. Paris: Asselin and Houzeau; 1878.
14. Marmor L. An unusual fracture of the tibial epiphysis. Clin Orthop Relat Res 1970; 73: 132–135.
15. Lynn MD. The triplane distal tibial epiphyseal fracture. Clin Orthop Relat Res 1972; 86: 187–190.
16. Dias LS, Giegerich CR. Fractures of the distal tibial epiphysis in adolescents. J Bone Joint Surg Am 1983; 65: 439–433.
17. Whipple TL, Martin DR, McIntyre LF, et al. Arthroscopic treatment of triplane fractures of the ankle. Arthroscopy 1993; 9: 456–463.
18. Jennings MM, Lagaay P, Schuberth JM. Arthroscopic assisted fixation of juvenile intra-articular epiphyseal ankle fractures. Foot Ankle Surg 2007; 46: 376–386.
19. Von Laer L. Classification, diagnosis, and treatment of transitional fractures of the distal part of the tibia. J Bone Joint Surg Am 1985; 67: 687–698.
20. Feldman DS, Otsuka NY, Hedden DM. Extra-articular triplane fractures of the distal tibial epiphysis. J Pediatr Orthop 1995; 15: 479–481.
21. Shin AY, Moran ME, Wenger DR. Intramalleolar triplane fractures of the distal tibial epiphysis. J Pediatr Orthop 1997; 17: 352–355.
22. Petit P, Panuel M, Faure F. Acute fracture of the distal tibial physis: role of gradient-echo MR imaging versus plain film examination. Am J Roentgenol 1996; 166: 1203–1206.
23. Kärrholm J, Hansson LI, Laurin S. Computer tomography of intraarticular supination-eversion fractures of the ankle in adolescents. J Pediatr Orthop 1981; 1: 181–187.
24. Cooperman DR, Spiegel PG, Laros GS. Tibial fractures involving the ankle in children. J Bone Joint Surg Am 1978; 60: 1040–1046.
25. Rapariz JM, Ocete G, Gonzalez-Herranz P, et al. Distal tibial triplane fractures: long term follow-up. J Pediatr Orthop 1996; 16: 113–118.
26. Imeda S, Takao M, Nishi H. Arthroscopically-assisted reduction and percutaneous fixation for triplane fracture of the distal tibia. Arthroscopy 2004; 20: e123–128.
27. McGillion S, Jackson M, Lahoti O. Arthroscopically assisted percutaneous fixation of triplane fractures of the distal tibia. J Pediatr Orthop Part B 2007; 16: 313–316.
28. Vahvanen V, Westerlund M, Nikku R. Lateral ligament injury of the ankle in children. Follow-up results of primary surgical treatment. Acta Orthop Scand 1984; 55: 21–25.
29. Haraguchi N, Kato F, Hayashi H. New radiographic projections for avulsion fractures of the lateral malleolus. J Bone Joint Surg Br 1998; 80: 684–688.
30. Danielsson LG. Avulsion fracture of the lateral malleolus in children. Injury 1989; 12: 165–167.
31. Busconi BD, Pappas AM. Chronic, painful ankle instability in skeletally immature athletes. Ununited osteochondral fractures of the distal fibula. Am J Sports Med 1996; 24: 647–651.

Chapter 14

Fractures and Dislocations of the Foot

Francisco Fernandez Fernandez

Introduction

Ninety percent of all fractures of the foot occur in the metatarsals and phalanges. Fractures of the tarsal bones are rare and have an incidence of about 4%.

The child's foot has a different growth pattern to other parts of the body. Fifty percent of the total growth in length is present by 1 year in girls and 18 months in boys. Ninety-six percent of the total growth is present by 12 years in girls and 88% in boys [1]. This pattern of growth must be considered when treating injuries of the foot in children [2, 3].

Talus

Epidemiology

The reported incidence of talar fractures is 0.08% of all fractures in children [4]. However, with increasing numbers of children participating in high velocity sports the incidence of fractures of the talus is increasing.

Mechanism of Injury

Axial trauma is the most common mechanism of fracture of the talus. It can also be the result of a direct crushing injury [5].

Blood Circulation

A major problem in talar fractures is the nature of the blood supply of the tarsal bone. Three-fifths of the talar surface is covered with cartilage and the main blood supply is through the non-cartilage covered talar neck. There is a centripetal blood supply via the sinus and tarsal canal [5]. The tarsal canal branch of the posterior tibial artery supplies the neck and the body of the talus. The sinus tarsi artery supplies blood to the head and lateral third of the talus. As a result fractures of the neck and proximal part of the talus carry a high risk of avascular necrosis.

Classification

Fractures of the talus are classified into those of the neck and those of the body, osteochondral fractures, and fractures of the posterior or lateral processes of the talus. In children fractures of the tarsal neck are the most frequent.

Fractures of the talar neck were classified according to Hawkins in 1970 into three types [6]. In this classification blood supply and the risk of avascular necrosis were taken into consideration. A rare type IV was added to the classification in 1978 by Canale and Kelly [7].

Modified Hawkins Classification of Talar Neck Fractures

- Type I: Fractures with no or minimal displacement. Only one source of blood supply entering through the talar neck may be disrupted.
- Type II: Displaced talar neck fracture with subluxation of the subtalar joint but no dislocation of the ankle joint. There may be a medial fracture with multiple fragments. At least two or three sources of blood supply may be damaged.
- Type III: Displaced talar neck fracture with dislocation of the body of the talus from the ankle with a subtalar joints. All three sources of blood supply likely to be damaged and a high risk of avascular necrosis.

F. Fernandez Fernandez (✉)
Department of Pediatric Orthopaedic Surgery, Olgahospital Stuttgart, Stuttgart, Germany

- Type IV: Displaced talar neck fracture with dislocation of the talar body from the ankle and subtalar joints associated with dislocation of the talar head and neck fragment from the talonavicular joint. All three sources of blood likely to be damaged and high risk of avascular necrosis.

Diagnosis

Clinically the foot and ankle are swollen and painful. There may be obvious deformity.

Standard anteroposterior (AP) and lateral radiographs of the ankle and foot should be taken. For further evaluation particularly if a fracture of the talus is suspected magnetic resonance imaging (MRI) or computed tomography (CT) can be helpful.

Treatment

Fracture of the Talar Neck

A Hawkins type I fracture without displacement should be immobilized in a below-knee leg cast.

A Hawkins type II fracture with medial comminution, displacement, and subtalar subluxation (Fig. 14.1) should be accurately fixed with a screw or K-wire. Open reduction via an anterolateral or anteromedial approach may be necessary. However, a postero-lateral approach avoids further risk to the blood supply.

Hawkins type III fractures must be treated as an emergency. Open reduction is mandatory. A closed reduction should not be attempted because of the limited chance of success and risk of further damage due to malrotation of the talar body and impingement on the tibialis posterior tendon. Open reduction should be performed with great care to avoid further damage to the blood supply. Stabilization should be obtained by screw fixation through a postero-lateral approach.

Hawkins type IV fractures should be treated as an emergency. Displacement of the neck of the talus, in addition to dislocation of the body, makes treatment of this fracture difficult. There is significant soft tissue injury and an even higher risk of avascular necrosis. The stabilization should be done by the postero-lateral approach. Screw fixation and temporary stabilization of the talonavicular joint for 4 weeks with a K-wire is the treatment of choice.

Fractures of the Body (Dome) of the Talus

Fractures of the body of the talus are unusual in children. The mechanism of injury is axial trauma. If the joint surface is damaged, open or arthroscopic reduction is advised.

Fractures of the Head of Talus

Fractures of the talar head are rare injuries (Fig. 14.2). They are often associated with complex injuries of the foot. In addition to cartilage damage, there are often defects of the

Table 14.1 Modified Hawkins classification of talar neck fractures, treatment, and risk of avascular necrosis (Canale and Kelly, 1978)

Type	Description	Treatment	Risk of osteonecrosis (%)
Type I	Undisplaced vertical fractures of the neck	Closed/open reduction	0–10
Type II	Displaced talar neck fracture with subtalar subluxation	Open/closed reduction	20–50
Type III	Displaced talar neck fracture, dislocation of the ankle and subtalar joints	Open emergency reduction	80–100
Type IV	Displaced talar neck fracture, dislocation of ankle, subtalar, and talonavicular joints	Open emergency reduction	90–100

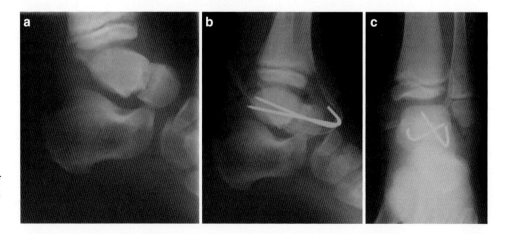

Fig. 14.1 (**a**) Six-year-old boy with a Hawkins type II fracture of the talar neck. (**b**) Open reduction and cross-pinning with Kirschner wires

Fig. 14.2 (**a**) Radiograph of a 10-year-old boy who had fallen from a bicycle and sustained a displaced fracture of the talar head and an infraction of the cuboid. (**b**) Closed reduction of the talar head and cross-pinning with K-wires

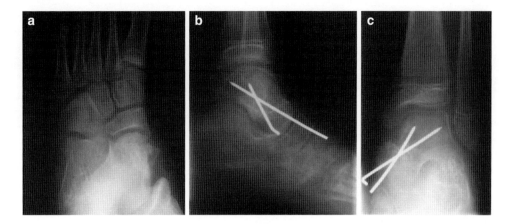

cancellous bone marrow. The aim of surgery is to restore the shape of the talar head and reestablish the medial column.

Fractures of the Lateral Talar Process

Fractures of the lateral talar process are sometimes overlooked or misdiagnosed. With the increase in sports such as snowboarding this injury is becoming more common. The mechanism of injury is dorsiflexion and inversion of the hindfoot. In non-displaced fractures conservative treatment is recommended. Displaced fractures affecting the joint should be reduced and fixed to avoid later joint degeneration [8, 9].

Calcaneus

Epidemiology

The incidence of calcaneus fractures in children varies between 0.05 and 0.15% of all fractures in children [10–12]. The incidence increases with the age and is highest in adolescence [13]. The developing calcaneus is largely cartilaginous, which is one of the reasons for the low incidence. Delayed diagnosis is reported in 43% of children with extraarticular fractures [14]. Some unrecognized calcaneal fractures in infants may be explained by their low morbidity and rapid healing.

Mechanism of Injury

The mechanism of injury depends on the child's age. Wiley and Profitt [14] describe falls from a height in children under the age of 10 years and high velocity injuries in children older than 10 and in adolescents. Atkins et al. [15] found a correlation between the height of the fall and the grade of injury in adults but this was not observed in children. Twenty to thirty percent of all fractures of the calcaneus in childhood are accompanied by other fractures. In the case of falls from a great height multiple injuries affecting the foot, the lower extremity, or the spine have to be considered. Two associated spinal injuries were found in 34 children with calcaneal fractures [14]. Associated injury to the soft tissues, nerves, and vessels is common [13, 16]. If a compartment syndrome is suspected emergency decompression should be performed (Fig. 14.3).

Classification and Clinical Appearance

Classifications of fractures of the calcaneus in children [13, 14] are shown in Table 14.2 and Fig. 14.4. Foot and ankle are swollen with abrasions or compression marks on the skin.

Imaging

Radiography

Anteroposterior and lateral views of the foot and ankle together with an axial view of the calcaneus should be taken.

It is important to look closely at the posterior facet of the calcaneus. In small children diagnosis can be difficult, in a toddler with a limp the fracture can be overlooked unless an axial view is taken. A follow-up radiograph 10 days after injury may show callus formation. A comparative view of the contralateral side can be helpful in these circumstances.

Fig. 14.3 Five-year-old boy who fell from a height sustaining a fractureture of the calcaneus in both feet. (**a**) *Top* and (**b**) *Bottom* calcaneus. Following treatment in closed casts in a primary care center he developed bilateral compartment syndrome. After delayed recognition of the compartment syndrome in both feet with major soft tissue necrosis and extensive osteonecrosis of both feet reconstruction with a latissimus dorsi flap was necessary

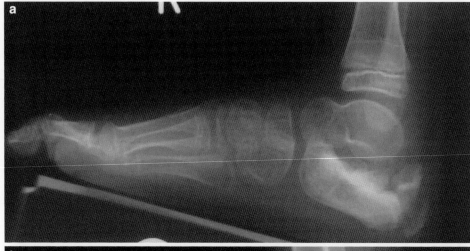

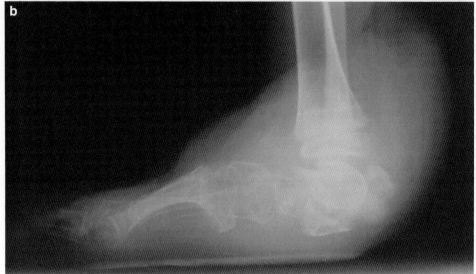

Table 14.2 Fractures of the calcaneus in children

Type I	a. Fracture of the tuberosity or apophysis
	b. Fracture of the sustentaculum
	c. Fracture of the anterior process
	d. Fracture of anterior inferolateral process
	e. Avulsion fracture of the body
Type II	Fracture of posterior and/or superior part of the tuberosity
Type III	Fracture of the body not involving the subtalar joint
Type IV	Fracture through the subtalar joint without displacement
Type V	Displaced fracture through the subtalar joint
Type VI	Fracture with serious soft tissue injury and bone loss

between 2 and 3 mm allow a three-dimensional reconstruction, however, the radiation dose must always be considered (see Chapter 5 of General Principles of Children's Orthopaedic Disease).

Magnetic Resonance Imaging

If available MRI is helpful to clarify the details of a fracture.

CT Scan

If an intraarticular fracture is suspected a CT scan is indicated to recognize the precise geometry and displacement of the fracture. To facilitate planning of the operation slices

Treatment

The aim of treatment is to restore the bony anatomy and to achieve a pain-free, functional, weight bearing, plantigrade foot.

is applied for 4–6 weeks. Weight bearing is allowed after 4 weeks.

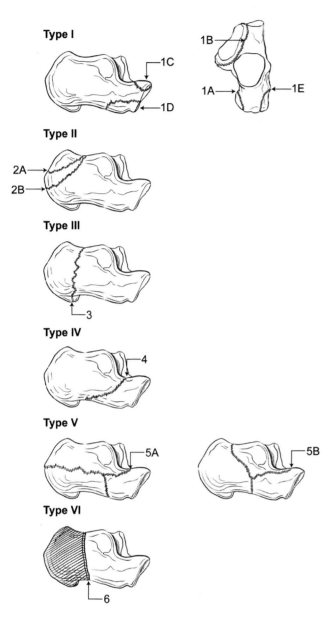

Fig. 14.4 Classification of fractures of the calcaneus

Undisplaced Fractures of the Calcaneus

In the past conservative treatment was the treatment of choice even for intraarticular fractures. Nowadays this is controversial. There is consensus regarding the management of extraarticular fractures. In non-displaced or minimally displaced extraarticular fractures immobilization in a split below-knee cast or a below-knee splint is indicated. As soon as the swelling subsides a complete below-knee cast

Displaced Fractures of the Calcaneus

Treatment of displaced intraarticular fractures is controversial. The published reports have low patient numbers and are retrospective case–control studies (level III for evidence). In two of these long-term studies good outcomes were reported following conservative treatment [17, 18]. In another study, 17 out of 19 fractures of the calcaneus treated conservatively and followed up for 17 years had excellent results [19].

In contrast to this conservative approach, open reduction has been advocated for displaced intraarticular fractures in children [20–22]. Depending on the pattern of fracture a semi-open or open reduction should be performed. When there is a depressed area of the posterior facet with only one fragment, reduction may be performed by a semi-open technique. A Steinmann pin is inserted into the calcaneus carefully avoiding the apophysis. Via an incision 1 cm below the displaced posterior facet a pusher screw is introduced. The pin is used to correct the shortening and varus deformity, the pusher screw straightens the displaced posterior facet and the percutaneous K-wires stabilize the intraarticular surface. The K-wires are left in situ for 4–6 weeks.

When there is a comminuted fracture of the posterior facet open reduction and internal fixation with a titanium plate are recommended (Fig. 14.5).

Fractures of the Midtarsal Bones

Injuries of the midfoot area are rare in children due to the relative shortness of the midtarsal bones and low body weight. The most common mechanism of injury is a crushing injury or direct force during a vehicle accident. Fractures of the midtarsal bones are often associated with injuries to the tarsometatarsal joint (so called Lisfranc joint) or the talonavicular/calcaneocuboid joint(so-called Chopart joint).

Fractures of the Navicular

Fractures of the navicular bone are rare and associated subluxation or dislocation is uncommon (Fig. 14.6). They are sometimes associated with displacement of the talonavicular/calcaneocuboid (Chopart) joint. Forced supination of the forefoot is thought to be the cause of this displacement. The aim of the treatment is to restore the medial and lateral columns using K-wire fixation. The blood supply to the navicular comes from the medial cuneiform and the talus. Variations in the appearance of the ossification center can be mistaken for a fracture particularly when associated with

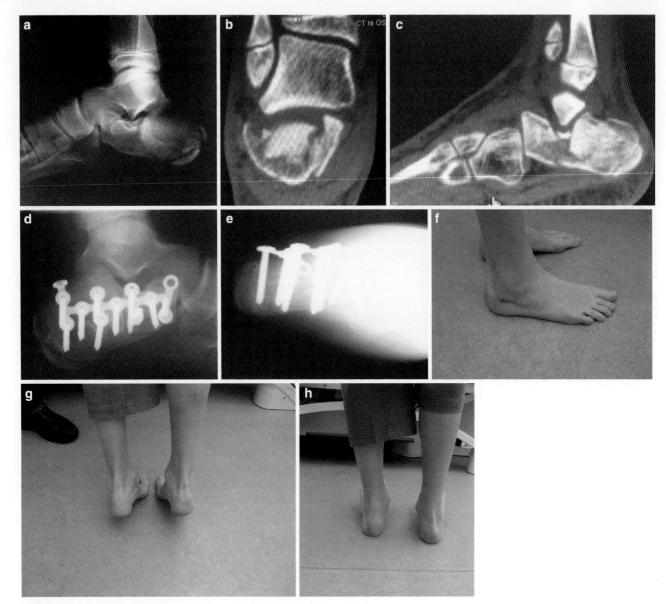

Fig. 14.5 (**a**) Thirteen-year-old boy with a comminuted fracture of the calcaneus. (**b** and **c**) There is considerable shortening and varus deformity on the CT scan. Multiple fragments with a considerable displacement of the posterior joint facet. (**d** and **e**) Open reduction and fixation using a plate. (**f**, **g** and **h**) Clinical picture 11/2 years after fracture. The patient has fully recovered and plays soccer

pain and local swelling as in osteochondritis of the tarsal navicular (Köhler's disease) (see Chapter 9 of Children's Upper and Lower Limb Orthopaedic Disorders) which is typically seen between the ages of 3 and 7 years.

Fractures of the Cuboid and Cuneiform Bones

The rare fractures of the cuboid are caused by compression. Fractures of the cuboid and cuneiform bones may be associated with dislocation of the Chopart joint. Compression force may cause shortening of the lateral column of the foot. Open or semi-open reduction and K-wire fixation is the treatment of choice.

Tarsometatarsal Injuries

Fracture/Dislocations of the Talonavicular/Calcaneocuboid (Chopart) and Tarsometatarsal (Lisfranc) Joints

Fracture/dislocations of the Chopart and Lisfranc joints are rare in childhood [23, 24]. The incidence in adults is between 0.02 and 0.9% of all fractures [25, 26]. Injuries of the Lisfranc joint are more common than those of the Chopart joint. In children these injuries are even less frequent.

Fig. 14.6 Ten-year-old gril following an injury on a sledge compression fracture of the navicular bone. Treatment in a below-knee cast for 6 weeks

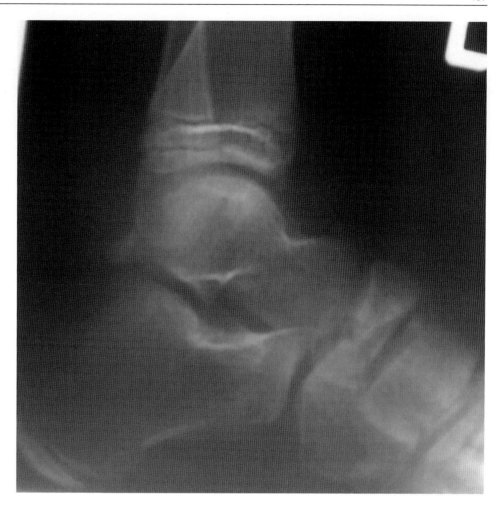

Mechanism of Injury

Fracture/dislocations of the Lisfranc joint are caused by a fall with the foot in a fixed plantarflexed position, a crush injury in a kneeling child, or being run over by a vehicle. The injury is associated with considerable soft tissue damage. The causes of injury to the Chopart joint are falls from a great height, or being run over by motor vehicles (Fig. 14.7)[27].

Classification of Lisfranc Fracture Dislocation

Fracture/dislocations of the Lisfranc joint were classified in 1909 by Quenu and Küss [28]. Zwipp [29] has suggested the following classification for tarsometatarsal fracture/dislocations:

1. Transligamental
2. Transcalcaneal
3. Transcuboidal
4. Transnavicular
5. Transtalar
6. Combination of injuries

Imaging

Three standard radiographic views are suggested for suspected Lisfranc injuries: a true lateral of the foot, a dorsoplantar view of the foot with a caudocranial angle of the X-ray tube of 20°, and a 45° angular view. If there is any doubt concerning a fracture/dislocation of the Lisfranc joint, a CT scan is advised.

For a Chopart joint injury again three views are suggested: a dorsoplantar view with the tube flexed 30°, a 45° angular view, and a true lateral view of the foot. Due to overlap of the tarsal bones interpretation can be difficult and if available, a CT scan is useful.

Treatment

In fracture/dislocation of the Lisfranc joint, the medial and lateral columns and the arch of foot should be reconstructed. The joint has suffered complex bone and ligament injury. If unrecognized and untreated, displacement of the Lisfranc joint produces malalignment of the mid and forefoot, which

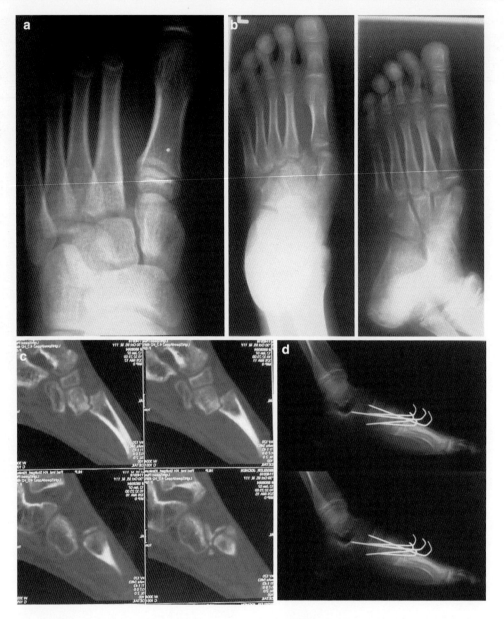

Fig. 14.7 **a**) Eleven-year-old boy with a divergent type Lisfranc fracture. (**b**) The diagnosis of a divergent Lisfranc fracture was not made until 2 months later. (**c**) The CT scans show the extent of the injury including fragmentation of the metatarsal base. (**d**) After open reduction of the fracture and K-wire fixation

causes considerable pain and discomfort. An anatomical reduction should be obtained if possible. If there is instability and a tendency to redisplace, percutaneous K-wire fixation is necessary. The interposition of soft tissue can prevent closed reduction and necessitate open reduction. The key to both closed and open reduction is the second metatarsal bone. The base of the second metatarsal must be correctly aligned with the intermediate (second) cuneiform bone.

Fracture/dislocations of the Chopart joint can be treated conservatively but if closed reduction fails open reduction is necessary followed by transarticular K-wire fixation and cast immobilization for 4 weeks.

Fractures of the Metatarsals

Metatarsal fractures are the second most common injuries to the foot after fractures of the phalanges. Single fractures result from direct or indirect force, while multiple fractures are commonly due to bicycle spoke injuries, participating in sports, or by run over injuries [30].

Single fractures are often minimally displaced and can be treated conservatively. Multiple fractures when displaced up to $\frac{1}{2}$ the diameter of the shaft may also be treated conservatively.

Fig. 14.8 (a) Eleven-year-old girl with displaced metatarsal fractures II–IV after a fall from a bicycle. (b) Closed reduction and percutaneous K-wire fixation

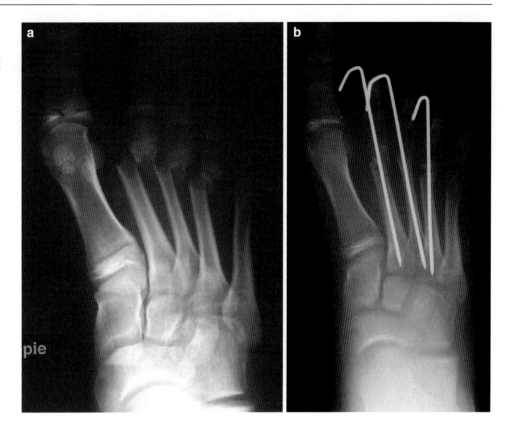

In children older than 10 years K-wire fixation may be indicated to ensure stability (Fig. 14.8).

Fracture of the Base of the Fifth Metatarsal

Mechanism of Injury

Fracture of the base of the fifth metatarsal is commonly caused by an inversion or rotational injury and can be mistaken for a sprained ankle particularly if the ankle and not the foot is radiographed (Fig. 14.9).

Classification

The classification is based on the localization of the fracture. Zone I is the area where the peroneus brevis and abductor digiti minimi tendons insert. Zone II begins distal to the tuberosity and includes the ligamentous attachments to the fourth metatarsal. Zone III is the proximal diaphyseal area.

The apophyseal growth center of the fifth metatarsal is oriented sagittally whereas most fractures of the base of the fifth metatarsal run transversally. This helps to differentiate the apophyseal growth center from a fracture.

Imaging

Two standard views (AP and oblique) are suggested for suspected fractures of the base of the fifth metatarsal. A lateral view is needed rarely.

Treatment

The treatment of a fracture of the base of the fifth metatarsal depends on displacement and zone.

In zone I most of the fractures are minimally displaced (not more than 2–3 mm) and they are avulsion fractures. Conservative treatment with a below-knee cast for 4–6 weeks is the treatment of choice. If the displacement is more than 2–3 mm an operative fixation is recommended.

Fractures in zone II and III are divided into stress fractures and acute injuries.

For stress fractures conservative treatment is usually satisfactory. However, if there is displacement of more than 2 mm operative stabilization with a tension-band technique may be necessary.

Acute injuries without displacement may be treated with a non-weight-bearing below-knee cast for 2–4 weeks followed

Fig. 14.9 (**a** and **b**) Thirteen-year-old girl with fracture of the base of fifth metatarsal after a bicycle accident, She had no treatment initially and presented with non-union 7 month later. (**c** and **d**) After resection of non-union and fixation with two screws

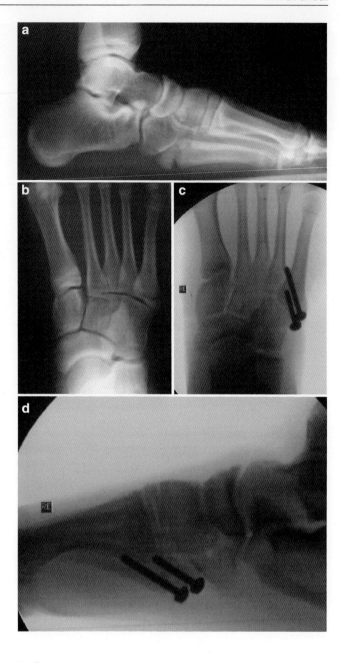

by 2 weeks in a walking cast. Again if there is displacement of more than 2 mm, surgical treatment is indicated.

Fractures of the Phalanges

Fractures of the toes (phalanges) are common. The usual mechanism of injury is crushing or direct injury to the toe. In the uncomplicated fracture taping to the neighboring uninjured toe for 2 weeks is sufficient. However, intraarticular fractures should be reduced and stabilized with one or two K-wires. Malunion should be avoided particularly in the first and fifth toes.

References

1. Anderson M, Blais MM, Green WT. Lengths of the growing foot. J Bone Joint Surg Am 1956; 38:998–1000.
2. De Valentine SJ. Epiphyseal injuries of the foot and ankle. Clin Pediatr Med Surg 1987; 4:279–310.
3. Silas SI, Herzenberg JE, Myerson MS, et al. Compartment syndrome of the foot in children. J Bone Joint Surg Am 1995; 77:356–361.
4. Höllwarth ME , Hausbrand D. Verletzungen der unteren Extremität. Das Verletzte Kind. Sauer (ed.) Stuttgart: Thieme; 1984.
5. Linhart WE, Höllwarth M. Talusfrakturen bei Kindern. Unfallchirurg 1985; 88:168–174.
6. Hawkins LG. Fractures of the neck of the talus. J Bone Joint Surg Am 1970; 52:991–1002.

7. Canale ST, Kelly FB Jr. Fractures of the neck of the Talus: long-term evaluation of seventy-one cases. J Bone Joint Surg Am 1978; 60:143–156.

8. Leibner ED, Symanovsky N, Abu-Sneinah K, et al. Fractures of the lateral process of the talus in children. J. Pediatr Orthop 2001; 10:68–72.

9. Noble J, Royle SG. Fracture of the lateral process of the talus: computed tomographic diagnosis. Br J Sports Med 1993; 26:245–246.

10. Van Frank E, Ward JC, Engelhardt P. Bilateral calcaneal fracture in children: case report and review of the literature. Arch Orthop Trauma Surg 1998; 118:11–112.

11. Thermann H, Schratt HE, Hüfner T, et al. Frakturen des kindlichen Fußes. Unfallchirurg 1998; 101:2–11.

12. Jarvis JG, Moroz PJ. Fractures and dislocations of the foot. In: Beaty JH, Kasser JR, eds. Rockwood and Wilkins' Fractures in Children, 6th ed. Philadelphia: Lippincott Williams & Wilkins; 2006.

13. Schmidt TL, Weiner DS. Calcaneal fractures in children. An evaluation of the nature of the injury in 56 children. Clin Orthop Relat Res 1982; 171:150–156.

14. Wiley JJ, Profitt A. Fractures of the os calcis in children. Clin Orthop Relat Res 1984; 188:131–138.

15. Atkins RM, Allen PE, Livingstone JA. Demographic features of intra-articular fractures of the calcaneum. Foot Ankle Surg 2001; 7:77–84.

16. Wiley JJ. Tarso-metatarsale joint injuries in children. J Pediatr Orthop 1981; 1:255–260.

17. Schantz K, Rasmussen F. Good prognosis after calcaneal fracture in childhood. Acta Orthop Scand 1988; 59:560–563.

18. Mora S, Thordarson DB, Zionts LE, et al. Pediatric calcaneal fractures. Foot Ankle Int 2001; 22:471–477.

19. Brunet JA. Calcaneal fractures in children. J Bone Joint Surg Br 2000; 82:211–216.

20. Inokuchi S, Usami N, Hiraishi E, et al. Calcaneal fractures in children. J Pediatr Orthop 1998; 18:469–474.

21. Ceccareli F, Faldini C, Piras F. Surgical versus non-surgical treatment of calcaneal fractures in children: a long-term results comparative study. Foot Ankle Int 2000; 21:825–832.

22. Buckinham R, Jackson M, Atkins R. Calcaneal fractures in adolescents. CT classification and results of operative treatment. Injury 2003; 34:454–459.

23. Kay RM, Tang CW. Pediatric foot fractures: evaluation and treatment. J AM Acad Orthop Surg 2003; 9:308–319.

24. Ribbans WJ, Natarajan R, Avala S. Pediatric foot fractures. Clin Orthop Relat Res 2005; 432:107–115.

25. Randt T, Dahlen C, Schikore H, et al. Dislocations fractures in the area of the middle foot-injuries of the Chopart and Lisfranc joint. Zentralbl Chir 1998; 123:1257–1266.

26. Jonson GF. Pediatric Lisfranc injury: "Bunk bed" fracture. AJR Am J Roentgenol 1981; 137:1041–1044.

27. Hosking KV, Hoffman EB. Midtarsal dislocations in children. J Pediatr Orthop 1999; 19:592–595.

28. Quenu E, Kuess G. Etude sur les luxations du metatarse (luxations metatarso-tarsiennes) du diastasis entre le ler et la 2e metatarsien. Rev Chir Orthop 1909; 39:281–336.

29. Zwipp H. Chirurgie des Fußes, Wien, New York: Springer; 1994.

30. Owen RJT, Hickey FG, Finlay DB. A study of metatarsal fractures in children. Injury 1995; 26:537–538.

Index

Printed by Printforce, the Netherlands